Basic Physics and
Measurement in Anaesthesia

Commissioning Editor: Paul Fam
Project Development Manager: Joanne Scott
Project Manager: Glenys Norquay
Illustration Manager: Michael J Ruddy
Design Manager: Andy Chapman
Illustrator: Tim Loughhead

Basic Physics and Measurement in Anaesthesia

Fifth Edition

P D Davis BSc DipAdvStSc CPhys MInstP MIPEM SRCS

Principal Physicist
Department of Clinical Physics and Bioengineering
Southern General Hospital
Glasgow

G N C Kenny BSc (Hons) MD FRCA FANZCA

Professor and Head
University Department of Anaesthesia
University of Glasgow

BUTTERWORTH
HEINEMANN

An Imprint of Elsevier Science

EDINBURGH LONDON NEW YORK OXFORD PHILADELPHIA ST LOUIS SYDNEY TORONTO 2003

Butterworth-Heinemann
An imprint of Elsevier Science Limited

First edition 1982
Second edition 1985
Third edition 1990
Reprinted 1991, 1992 (twice), 1993, 1994
Fourth edition 1995
Reprinted 1995, 1996, 1997, 1998 (twice), 1999, 2000, 2001, 2002 (twice)

© G D Parbrook, P D Davis and E O Parbrook, 1982, 1985, 1990
© P D Davis, G D Parbrook and G N C Kenny, 1995

ISBN 0 7506 4828 7

British Library Cataloguing in Publication Data
A catalogue record for this book is available from the British Library

Library of Congress Cataloging in Publication Data
A catalog record for this book is available from the Library of Congress

Note
Medical knowledge is constantly changing. Standard safety precautions must be followed, but as new research and clinical experience broaden our knowledge, changes in treatment and drug therapy may become necessary or appropriate. Readers are advised to check the most current product information provided by the manufacturer of each drug to be administered to verify the recommended dose, the method and duration of administration, and contraindications. It is the responsibility of the practitioner, relying on experience and knowledge of the patient, to determine dosages and the best treatment for each individual patient. Neither the Publisher nor the editors/contributors assumes any liability for any injury and/or damage to persons or property arising from this publication.

ELSEVIER
SCIENCE
your source for books,
journals and multimedia
in the health sciences
www.elsevierhealth.com

The
publisher's
policy is to use
**paper manufactured
from sustainable forests**

Printed in China

Contents

Preface to First Edition

Our aim is to provide sufficient understanding of physics and its clinical application to allow the practising anaesthetist to give safe and reliable anaesthesia. In addition, this book should help to bridge the gap between the level of teaching in school and in undergraduate curricula and that in the more advanced textbooks on clinical physics. It is not intended to provide a rigorous treatment of physics or to act as a detailed reference text; consequently, references have been omitted. The use of mathematics, too, has been strictly limited and to render the subject more interesting to anaesthetists clinical examples are sometimes provided in detail, even though this may involve digression into the realms of physiology and clinical anaesthesia.

Although written with the needs of the anaesthetist in mind, we hope the book may also be of interest to technical and senior nursing staff working in the operating theatre and intensive care areas.

Measurement is an integral part of physics and is included in the book because monitoring equipment plays such an important part in clinical anaesthesia. Nevertheless, all aspects of clinical measurement are not covered and details of physiological, biochemical and haematological measurement are not provided.

Previous experience in preparing an audiotape-slide series on *Clinical Physics and Measurement for Anaesthetists* has been helpful in the preparation of this book, but the content of the work is not identical with that of the audiovisual series and is so designed that it may be used either on its own or to complement the series.

The SI system of units is used throughout, and a resumé of the definitions of these units of measurement is given in the Appendix. The exponent is used instead of the solidus because this is the more common form.

We are grateful to colleagues for their help and in particular to Dr W G Anderson for assistance with the chapter on Oxygen Measurement and to Dr R. Hughes for advice on the chapters on Blood Pressure Measurement and on Measurement of pH and CO_2. We are also grateful to Mr I B Monk for help with much of the original material.

We should also like to thank Mr B D Cameron, our graphic designer, for his expert production of the diagrams for this book.

G D Parbrook
P D Davis
E O Parbrook

1982

Preface to Fifth Edition

Since the publication of the first edition, equipment for use in anaesthesia has become ever more complex. More new applications of physical principles have been introduced since the fourth edition of this book, so a fifth edition has been prepared. As before, references to older equipment that is not in current use have been retained where these are important in the demonstration of physical principles or where they are of historical significance.

For this edition, Dr G D Parbrook has finally retired from authorship. The remaining authors wish to acknowledge his enormous contribution over the years, which has formed the foundation for this current volume.

P D Davis
G N C Kenny

Pressure

Introduction, Force

As the anaesthetist makes pressure measurements both in patients and on the anaesthetic machine, an understanding of this topic is essential. Before concentrating on pressure, however, the definition of force must be considered. Force is that which changes or tends to change the state of rest or motion of an object. In the SI system (see Appendix), force is measured in newtons (N), a newton being the force that will give a mass of 1 kilogram an acceleration of 1 metre per second per second.

$$N = kg\ m\ s^{-2}$$

The force of gravity acting on any object will give the object an acceleration of $9.81\ m\ s^{-2}$. Therefore, the force of gravity on a mass of 1 kilogram must be 9.81 N. This force is known as 1 kilogram weight, so 1 newton is equivalent to $\frac{1}{9.81}$ kilogram weight, i.e. 102 gram weight.

Pascals, Bars

Pressure is the force applied or distributed over a surface, and is expressed as force per unit area. The SI unit of pressure is the pascal (Pa) and 1 pascal is a pressure of 1 newton acting over an area of 1 square metre. As the weight of 102 grams acting over 1 square metre represents a tiny pressure, the unit of pressure commonly used is not the pascal, but the kilopascal (kPa). For high-pressure gas supplies, the bar is used as the unit. Although it is not an SI unit, it has been retained for general use. One bar equals 100 kilopascals and is also the approximate atmospheric pressure at sea level. Consequently, the gauge pressure of 137 bar in a full oxygen cylinder is equivalent to about 137 atmospheres. The interrelationship of bars and atmospheres is considered further in Chapter 4.

The Interrelationship of Pressure and Force

It is easier to understand pressure and force in the context of examples taken from anaesthetic practice.

Figure 1.1 illustrates the relative difficulty of injecting a liquid from a large and from a small syringe. The pressure developed in the syringe depends on the force and the area over which it is applied.

$$P = \frac{f}{a}$$

where P is the pressure, f is the force and a is the area.

Figure 1.1 Effect of doubling syringe diameter on the pressure which is generated

If the force exerted by the thumb is similar for the two syringes, the pressure available for injection is greatly increased by the small area of the plunger of the small syringe because this pressure is inversely proportional to the cross-sectional area of the plunger. If this area is increased by a factor of four by doubling the syringe diameter, the pressure generated is reduced by a factor of four, provided that the force on the plunger is the same.

Thumb pressure on the end of a syringe plunger can produce a force of 25 newtons. If the area of the plunger in a 2 ml syringe is 5×10^{-5} square metres, the pressure generated in the syringe is as follows:

$$\frac{25 \text{ N}}{5 \times 10^{-5} \text{ m}^2} = 500 \text{ kPa}$$

The pressure of 500 kPa is approximately five times atmospheric pressure, so it is easy to produce extravascular infusion unintentionally with such a syringe.

The area of the plunger of a 20 ml syringe is greater, e.g. 2.5×10^{-4} square metres, so a similar calculation shows that a lower pressure of 100 kPa (about 1 atmosphere) may be produced. Nevertheless, this is still six times a typical systolic blood pressure of 16 kPa (120 mmHg). The pressure generated when local analgesic is injected from a 20 ml syringe can give rise to accidents during a technique known as intravenous regional analgesia. In this technique a blood pressure cuff inflated above systolic pressure is used to protect the patient from the systemic effects of local analgesic injected into a distal vein. From the calculations already given, it can be seen that pressures in the vein during rapid injection can exceed the systolic pressure, so the protection from the blood pressure cuff can be inadequate, particularly if a vein adjacent to the cuff is used.

Some syringe pumps and infusion pumps can also generate high pressures, so care should be taken to ensure that cannulae are correctly placed and that extravascular infusion does not occur.

Another clinical example of pressure generated by force acting over an area is the formation of bed sores in an immobilized patient. Suppose 20 kg of the patient's weight are supported by an area of contact between the patient and the bed of 10^{-2} square metres (an area equal to 10 cm × 10 cm). The force over this area is:

$$20 \text{ kg} \times 9.81 \text{ m s}^{-2} = 196 \text{ N}$$

The pressure is therefore:

$$\frac{196 \text{ N}}{10^{-2} \text{ m}^2} = 19.6 \text{ kPa}$$

A typical systolic blood pressure is only 16 kPa, so the blood supply to this area is cut off and there is a risk of ischaemia and bed sores at this pressure point.

Figure 1.2 Pressure relief valve

Spring exerting force f

Disc area a

Pressure P

Pressure relief valves and expiratory valves of anaesthetic breathing systems also provide simple examples of the balance between force and pressure exerted over an area.

As shown in Fig. 1.2, the pressure P inside an anaesthetic breathing system acts over the area a of the disc of an expiratory valve to exert a force. If this force is greater than the force f exerted by the spring, the disc rises to release gas. In the case of the expiratory valve, a very light spring is used so that low pressures (e.g. 50 Pa) suffice to open the valve at its minimum setting, but an anaesthetist can raise the pressure by screwing down the cap above the spring if required.

In the safety valve found on most anaesthetic machines, a stronger spring is used so that the pressure cannot rise above about 35 kPa and damage the component parts of the machine. A similar safety valve is incorporated into ventilators but is set to a lower level (e.g. 7 kPa).

Pressure-reducing valves, also known as pressure regulators, are used in anaesthetic machines to reduce the pressure and control the supply of gas from the cylinders. These valves also work by balancing the force of a spring against that from the pressure on a diaphragm.

In the pressure-reducing valve illustrated in Fig. 1.3, as the low pressure P_2 falls, the force acting on the diaphragm from below falls and the spring pushes the diaphragm down. When the diaphragm descends it carries with it a rod connected to a small valve which controls the supply of gas at high pressure P_1 and so maintains the pressure P_2 in the compartment below the diaphragm at its correct level.

Figure 1.3 shows a single-stage reducing valve, but two-stage valves are also available.

Figure 1.4 shows an Entonox valve, a two-stage valve in which the first stage is identical to the reducing valve described above. The flow of gas from the outlet of the second-stage valve is controlled by a large diaphragm 'd'. Movements of this diaphragm tilt a rod, which regulates the flow of the gas out of the first-stage

Figure 1.3 Pressure reducing valve

Spring force f

Diaphragm area a

High-pressure inlet P_1

Low-pressure outlet P_2

Figure 1.4 Entonox valve, illustrating the first-stage and second-stage pressure reducing valves

valve. The second stage is adjusted so that gas flows only when the pressure is below atmospheric pressure. The Entonox valve is an example of a demand valve and similar valves are sometimes used by firemen in breathing apparatus and by aeroplane pilots for oxygen administration.

Control and warning mechanisms which are attached to the high-pressure oxygen supply in many anaesthetic machines operate on a similar principle to the reducing valve.

An example of an oxygen-failure warning device is illustrated in Fig. 1.5. When the oxygen supply pressure falls below a set minimum value, the force acting on the diaphragm fails to hold it against the spring. The diaphragm moves down and oxygen leaks past the small valve to blow the whistle, thereby giving a warning of the falling oxygen pressure.

A system of this type with a diaphragm and valve may also be used to cut off the nitrous oxide supply during an oxygen supply failure.

Gauge and Absolute Pressures

A full oxygen cylinder has a gauge pressure of 137 bar. When the cylinder is empty, the gauge records 0 bar but, unless a vacuum pump has been used, the cylinder still contains oxygen at the ambient atmospheric pressure, and the true or absolute pressure in the empty cylinder is about 1 bar (Fig. 1.6).

In most cases, anaesthetists can ignore atmospheric pressure and use gauges that record the gauge pressure above or below existing atmospheric pressure. Thus, ventilator and gas-cylinder pressures, arterial blood pressure and venous pressure readings are all gauge pressures.

To avoid confusion, the term 'absolute pressure' is used when the total pressure including atmospheric pressure is required. The absolute pressure for the empty oxygen cylinder is about 1 bar; so for a full cylinder, if the gauge pressure is 137 bar, the absolute pressure is 138 bar.

Absolute pressure = Gauge pressure + Atmospheric pressure

Figure 1.5 Oxygen failure warning device

Figure 1.6
Interrelationship of
gauge, atmospheric and
absolute pressure

Atmospheric pressure at the surface of the earth is due to the gravitational force on the air molecules above, the actual pressure depending on the density of air over the point concerned, which, in turn, depends on altitude and weather conditions.

Pressure in Liquids

In the same way that the gravitational force on the air molecules gives rise to atmospheric pressure, so the force of gravity on the molecules of a liquid gives rise to a pressure that depends on the height of liquid above the point of measurement. This is used as the measuring principle in instruments such as manometers and is normally independent of the cross-sectional area of the column of liquid used.

Figure 1.7 illustrates the pressures P_1 and P_2 at the bottom of 10.2 cm high water columns with cross-sectional areas of 1 cm^2 and 4 cm^2, respectively. The

Figure 1.7 Pressure at
the base of a column
of water

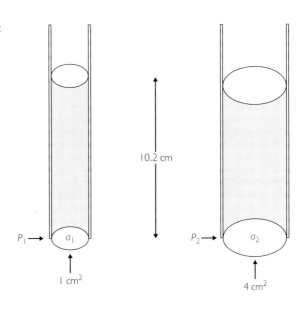

pressures P_1 and P_2 can be calculated if it is remembered that 10.2 cm^3 water weighs 10.2 g. Therefore:

$$P_1 = \frac{f_1}{a_2} = \frac{10.2\text{g wt}}{1\,\text{cm}^2} = 10.2 \text{ g wt cm}^{-2}$$

and

$$P_2 = \frac{f_2}{a_2} = \frac{4 \times 10.2\text{g wt}}{4 \text{ cm}^2} = 10.2 \text{ g wt cm}^{-2}$$

The example shows that the pressure in water at 10.2 cm depth will always be 10.2 g wt cm^{-2}. To convert the unorthodox figure of 10.2 g wt cm^{-2} into SI units the calculation is as follows:

Pressure of 10.2 cmH$_2$O = 10.2 g wt cm^{-2}

= 10.2×10^4 g wt m^{-2}

= 102 kg wt m^{-2}

Since 102 g wt = 1 N

Pressure of 10.2 cmH$_2$O = 1 kN m^{-2}

= 1 kPa

Hence 10.2 cm of water pressure is 1 kilopascal. In practice, however, most water manometers are still calibrated in centimetres of water pressure and are calibrated so that the height of the liquid column can be read directly.

Effect of Surface Tension

Although the pressure is normally unaffected by the diameter of the manometer tube, surface tension may influence the readings in narrow capillary tubes, increasing the reading in the case of a water manometer and decreasing it in a mercury manometer.

Figure 1.8 illustrates the molecular basis of surface tension. On the left, the diagram shows the forces of attraction which act on a molecule at some depth in a liquid and those which act on a molecule in the surface layer. In the surface layer, some of the forces of attraction between the molecules act in a direction parallel to the surface of the liquid and result in the liquid surface behaving as though a skin were present. This is the phenomenon known as surface tension. If all the forces between the molecules on either side of an imaginary straight line on the surface of the liquid are summed, the resulting surface tension may be expressed in terms of force per unit length (newtons per metre in SI units).

Figure 1.8 Molecular basis of surface tension

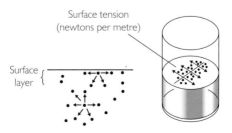

Figure 1.9 Effect of surface tension at a meniscus

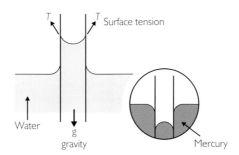

In addition to the forces of attraction between the molecules of a liquid, there are also forces between the molecules and the walls of the containing vessel. These forces result in the meniscus, the curvature of a liquid surface at its contact with the wall. Figure 1.9 shows a vertical glass capillary tube with its lower end immersed in water. Because of the meniscus, the surface tension (T) at the junction between the water and the wall of the tube acts to some extent in a vertical direction and pulls the water up the tube until it is balanced by the force of gravity on the water in the tube which is above the normal liquid level. The water rises up the capillary tube to a height that is inversely proportional to the radius of the tube.

In the case of mercury, a convex meniscus forms because the mercury does not wet the tube, so surface tension depresses the level of liquid in the capillary tube.

Effect of Slope in a Manometer Tube

If a manometer tube is tilted, the liquid rises along it until the necessary vertical height is achieved (Fig. 1.10). Particularly sensitive gauges sometimes use a sloped manometer tube and are appropriately calibrated, but in anaesthetic practice most manometer tubes are intended for vertical use.

Mercury Manometers

If a dense liquid such as mercury is used, a manometer may be used to measure higher pressures. Mercury is 13.6 times as dense as water, so the force exerted by its weight is proportionately greater. A pressure which supports a 7.5 mm column of mercury will support a 10.2 cm column of water (Fig. 1.11).

Figure 1.10 Effect of slope on manometer calibration

Figure 1.11 Comparison of water and mercury manometers

The pressures in the two manometers may be compared as follows:

Pressure exerted by 7.5 mmHg = 13.6×7.5 mmH$_2$O

= 10.2 cmH$_2$O

= 1 kPa

Mercury is useful in manometers measuring up to atmospheric pressure (1 bar or 100 kPa) and, as 1 kPa equals 7.5 mmHg, it is obvious that 1 bar is 750 mmHg pressure. The units of bar and kilopascal have the advantage that they are independent of changes of gravitational force and of temperature, which can affect the height of a mercury column.

It is essential that the top of a manometer tube is open. In the mercury manometers used for blood pressure measurements, a disc of material permeable to air is placed at the top of the tube to prevent spillage of the mercury, but this creates a potential problem in that dirt or grease may partially obstruct the disc, thus leading to faulty readings.

In contrast to the standard open-ended manometer tube used for gauge pressure, the mercury barometer used to measure atmospheric pressure is sealed, as shown in Fig. 1.12. A vacuum is present above the mercury so that the full absolute pressure is recorded.

As an alternative to a manometer, a Bourdon gauge (illustrated in Fig. 1.13) may be used. This type of pressure gauge is essential for the measurement of high pressures, where the required height of the fluid column in a manometer would be impractical. In the Bourdon gauge, increasing gas pressure causes a tube to uncoil and in doing so moves a pointer over a scale on a dial. Bourdon gauges have the advantage over manometers that there is no liquid to spill. They are also known as aneroid gauges from the Greek 'a-neros' (without liquid).

Figure 1.12
Mercury barometer

Figure 1.13
Bourdon gauge

Another form of aneroid gauge is based on a bellows or capsule which expands or contracts depending on the pressure across it. Two forms are illustrated in Fig. 1.14: the one on the left is sealed and is sensitive to changes of atmospheric or absolute pressure; the one on the right has the interior open to the surrounding air and is suitable for measuring gauge pressure.

Differential Pressure

In addition to absolute pressure and gauge pressure, differential pressure is sometimes measured. Differential pressure is the difference between two pressures, e.g. between two points in an anaesthetic breathing system. The aneroid gauge shown on the right of Fig. 1.14 can act as a differential gauge if connections are made at X and Y, i.e. to the inside and outside of the capsule.

Other Units

In this chapter the units pascal, bar, mmHg and cmH_2O have been used because these are the units encountered in anaesthetic practice. Units of pounds per square inch are also sometimes seen, 14.5 lb $inch^{-2}$ being 1 bar. Torr may be used on vacuum gauges; 7.5 torr is 1 kPa (1 torr is about 1 mmHg).

Figure 1.14 Types of bellows aneroid gauges

Fluid Flow

2

Flow is defined as the quantity of a fluid, i.e. a gas or liquid, passing a point in unit time:

$$F = \frac{Q}{t}$$

where F is the mean flow, Q is the quantity (mass or volume) and t is the time.

In this chapter, flow is represented by the rate of change of quantity to avoid the need to specify mass or volume. On graphs and illustrations the symbol $\dot{Q}$ is used, the small dot above the Q indicating rate of change of Q. The symbol Q without the dot stands for quantity.

Laminar Flow

In laminar flow (Fig. 2.1), a fluid moves in a steady manner and there are no eddies or turbulence. This is the type of flow normally present in smooth tubes at low rates of flow.

The flow is greatest in the centre, being about twice the mean flow, as illustrated by the longer arrows in the figure. As the side of the tube is approached, the flow becomes slower until it approaches zero at the wall. In order to drive a fluid through a tube, a pressure difference must be present across the ends.

The graph in Fig. 2.2 shows the result if various flows are passed through a tube and the resulting pressure drop across the ends is recorded. There is a linear relationship such that flow is directly proportional to pressure under conditions of laminar flow. The ratio of pressure to flow is a constant known as the resistance R of the apparatus or tube concerned.

Figure 2.3 shows how resistance can be measured. A known constant flow is passed through the apparatus concerned and the difference in pressure $P_1 - P_2$ between the ends of the apparatus is measured. By dividing the pressure difference by the flow the resistance of the apparatus is obtained and, provided that flow is laminar, the resistance is independent of the flow.

Figure 2.1 Laminar flow

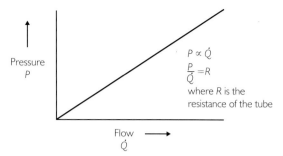

Figure 2.2 The linear relationship of flow to pressure in laminar flow

Figure 2.3 Measurement of flow resistance

A technique such as this may be used to measure resistance with either gas or liquid flow. Alternatively, for liquids, a constant head of pressure may be achieved by means of a reservoir of liquid and measurement of the resulting flow allows calculation of the resistance. A system of this type may be used to illustrate what happens if the diameter of a tube is halved (Fig. 2.4).

It is found that this reduction of the diameter has a pronounced effect on the resistance to flow. Halving the diameter reduces the flow to one-sixteenth of its original value if the pressure drop along the tube remains the same. In other words, the flow is proportional to the fourth power of the diameter. Consequently, a slight reduction of the diameter of an endotracheal tube can have an appreciable effect on resistance and therefore on flow.

As shown in Fig. 2.5, the effect of altering the length of the tube is much less marked than that of altering the diameter. If the length of the tube is halved, the flow will double, other factors being kept constant. Finally, the viscosity of the

Figure 2.4 Effect on flow of halving the tube diameter

Figure 2.5 Effect on flow of halving the length of a tube

fluid affects resistance to laminar flow in such a way that the flow decreases as the viscosity increases. Viscosity is a measure of the frictional forces acting between the layers of the fluid as it flows along the tube. It is represented by the Greek letter eta (η) and has the units of pascal seconds.

The effects described may be summarized as follows:

$$\dot{Q} \propto P$$

$$\propto d^4$$

$$\propto \frac{1}{l}$$

$$\propto \frac{1}{\eta}$$

where $\dot{Q}$ is the flow through the tube, P is the pressure across the tube, d is the diameter of the tube, l is the length of the tube and η is the viscosity of the fluid.

All these factors can be combined with a proportionality constant, $\pi/128$, in an equation which can be derived theoretically and is known as the Hagen–Poiseuille equation:

$$\dot{Q} = \frac{\pi P d^4}{128\eta l}$$

This equation can be rearranged to show how the pressure drop across a tube depends on various factors:

$$P = \frac{128\eta l \dot{Q}}{\pi d^4}$$

Turbulent Flow

Laminar flow is not the only type of flow occurring in anaesthetic apparatus, breathing systems, the airways and the circulation.

As illustrated in Fig. 2.6, laminar flow may change to turbulent flow if a constriction is reached which results in the fluid velocity increasing. In turbulent flow, fluid no longer flows in a smooth fashion but swirls in eddies and the resistance is higher than for the same laminar flow. The variation of fluid velocity across the tube is different in turbulent flow from that which occurs in laminar flow and the flow is no longer directly proportional to pressure.

Onset of Turbulent Flow

Although turbulent flow may occur if there is a sharp increase in the flow through a tube, there are several other factors influencing the type of flow, such as the

Figure 2.6 Onset of turbulent flow

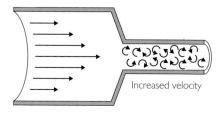

Increased velocity

viscosity and density of the fluid and the diameter of the tube. These factors may all be combined to give an index known as the Reynolds number, which is calculated as follows:

$$\text{Reynolds number} = \frac{v\rho d}{\eta}$$

where v is the linear velocity of the fluid, ρ is the density, d is the diameter of the tube and η is the viscosity.

Empirical measurements with cylindrical tubes show that, if the Reynolds number exceeds about 2000, then turbulent flow is likely to be present. If the Reynolds number is below 2000, the flow is likely to be laminar.

It can be seen from this formula that for a fixed set of conditions there is a critical velocity at which the Reynolds number has the value of 2000. When the velocity of the fluid exceeds this critical value, the character of the flow is likely to change from laminar to turbulent. This critical velocity applies only for a given fluid in a given tube. Turbulent flow is often present where there is an orifice, a sharp bend or some other irregularity which may cause a local increase in velocity and hence an increase in the Reynolds number to a value above 2000.

An example of the effect of density on the onset of turbulent flow is the use of helium in respiratory disorders. In this case, helium reduces the density of gas inhaled and so reduces the incidence of turbulent flow. A lower resistance to breathing results because the transition from turbulent to laminar flow is associated with a marked decrease in resistance to flow through a tube.

Characteristics of Turbulent Flow

The theoretical analysis of turbulent flow is highly complex and although it is possible to predict some aspects of flow behaviour, much of what is known has been learnt from experiments. As in the case of laminar flow, the flow through a tube is proportional to the pressure difference between the ends of the tube. Above a certain value of the Reynolds number, which decreases as the roughness of the inside of the tube increases, the pressure difference is proportional to the density of the fluid and the square of the flow. Under these circumstances, as shown in Fig. 2.7, in order to double the flow, the pressure must be increased by a factor of four. As the relationship of pressure to flow is no longer linear, resistance is not constant and when referring to resistance in the presence of turbulent flow, it is important that the flow at which the resistance is measured is specified. For example, the resistance to the flow of air during breathing depends on the air flow if the flow is turbulent.

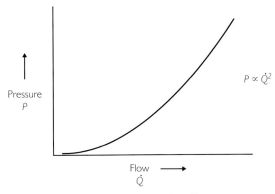

$P \propto \dot{Q}^2$

Pressure
P

Flow $\longrightarrow$
$\dot{Q}$

Figure 2.7 Relationship of flow to pressure in turbulent flow

The factors affecting flow and pressure during this type of turbulent flow are as follows:

$$\dot{Q} \propto \sqrt{P} \qquad P \propto \dot{Q}^2$$
$$\propto \frac{1}{\sqrt{l}} \qquad \propto l$$
$$\propto \frac{1}{\sqrt{\rho}} \qquad \propto \rho$$

where $\dot{Q}$ is the flow, P is the pressure across the tube, l is the length of the tube and ρ is the density of the fluid.

The property of the fluid passing through the tube that is important in turbulent flow is the density, which is represented by the Greek letter rho (ρ) and is equal to mass divided by volume ($kg\ m^{-3}$).

The pressure difference necessary to produce a given flow increases as the diameter of the tube decreases, the increase required being slightly greater than that for laminar flow. However it is not expressible as a simple power of the diameter.

For flow which is neither laminar nor for which the Reynolds number is above the appropriate value as discussed above, there is some dependence on viscosity as well as density. No simple formula can be given to relate pressure drop to other factors.

Clinical Aspects of Flow

Changes between laminar and turbulent flow depend on the velocity of the gas, which in turn depends on the volume flow and thus on the diameter of the tubing and airways. The flow at which transition takes place depends on the gases present. Figure 2.8 illustrates the critical flows for a typical anaesthetic mixture of 60% nitrous oxide in oxygen and also for air at an ambient temperature of 20°C. In the patient's airway, gases are humidified, contain carbon dioxide and are at a temperature of 34–37°C. The combined effect of these changes is a rise in critical flow due to the dominant effect of the reduction in density from the warming of the gases. Consequently, the critical flow for the humidified, warmed anaesthetic mixture in the patient could be 10% higher than the figures for dry gases at 20°C illustrated on the graph.

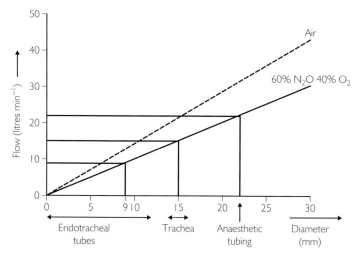

Figure 2.8 Critical flow in smooth tubes for air and for a mixture of 60% nitrous oxide and 40% oxygen. The values are for dry gas at 20°C and would be slightly higher for warmed humidified gas (see text)

As shown in Fig. 2.8, the critical flow in litres per minute for a typical anaesthetic gas has approximately the same numerical value as the diameter of the airway concerned in millimetres. Thus the flow of anaesthetic gases in a 9 mm internal diameter endotracheal tube becomes turbulent when flow exceeds about 9 litres min^{-1}, the flow in a 15 mm diameter trachea is turbulent at flows over 15 litres min^{-1}, whereas in the 22 mm internal diameter tubing of breathing systems, flow becomes turbulent when flows greater than 22 litres min^{-1} occur. As breathing is cyclical, with peak flows over 50 litres min^{-1}, turbulent flow usually predominates during peak flow, whereas laminar flow is present at other times in the respiratory cycle. As shown in Fig. 2.8, the critical flows for air are higher than those for a mixture of nitrous oxide and oxygen, so laminar flow prevails to a greater extent, especially in the wider breathing tubes.

Although the bronchi and smaller air passages in the lungs are even narrower than the trachea, the air flow through them is slower, so laminar flow is usual in the lower respiratory tract.

The 30 mm diameter indicated on the figure is also relevant in anaesthesia as this is the internal diameter of scavenging transfer tubing and is the size used in some respiratory equipment in which a low respiratory resistance is required.

The examples given assume that the tubes are smooth. The corrugated surface of anaesthetic tubing induces turbulence at a lower flow than a smooth tube. In addition, any sharp bends or angles increase the incidence of turbulent flow. As an example, Fig. 2.9 illustrates turbulence at the connector of an endotracheal tube.

In quiet breathing, the flow within the respiratory tract is principally laminar, but during speaking, coughing or deep breathing, turbulent flow tends to occur as the critical velocity is exceeded. In practice, many other factors can increase the likelihood of turbulent flow in the respiratory tract, e.g. a lining layer of mucus may affect the flow by narrowing the respiratory passages.

Similar considerations apply to the circulation, the flow being principally laminar, but with the possibility of turbulence at the junctions of vessels or where

Figure 2.9 Turbulent flow at an endotracheal tube connector

vessels are constricted by outside pressures. Turbulence in the circulatory system often results in a bruit which can be heard on auscultation.

The blood vessels and bronchi, however, are not rigid tubes but have a variable radius depending on the pressure gradient across their walls and on the tone of the elastic and smooth muscle tissue in their walls. The muscle tone affects the tension in the walls; these changes in tension alter the radius, thereby affecting the flow.

Tension

As shown in Fig. 2.10, tension is a tangential force in newtons per metre acting on a length of the wall A–B. A balance must be present between the pressure caused by the smooth muscle and elastic tissue and the fluid pressure in the tube in order to prevent the tube progressively distending or collapsing. The pressure caused by the tension of the smooth muscle and elastic tissue may be calculated from Laplace's law. For a tube, Laplace's law states:

$$\text{Pressure gradient across the wall of a tube} = \frac{\text{Tension}}{\text{Radius}}$$

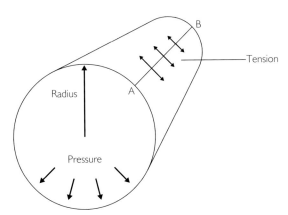

Figure 2.10 Relationship between pressure, radius and tension in a distensible tube

The application of this law shows a potential instability in the radius of vessels. A fall in pressure in an arteriole, for example, tends to distend it less and so could reduce its radius, but the smooth muscle in the wall maintains tension, so the ratio of tension to radius is increased and pressure across the wall is raised (Laplace's law). Instability then results with contraction and closure of the vessel. This can occur clinically at a low pressure known as the critical closing pressure for the vessel. Similarly, bronchioles and alveolar ducts may close when a critical closing pressure is present in the airways on expiration. For vessels and bronchi to remain patent, a correct balance between the pressures across their walls and the tensions from the elastic tissue and smooth muscle is essential. In addition to these sources of tension, surface tension is also present at air–liquid interfaces as explained in Chapter 1.

Surface Tension

The surface tension of the moisture present in alveoli and alveolar ducts can lead to potential instability. When the radius of the alveolar ducts and alveoli diminish during expiration, the pressure across the wall tends to rise (Laplace's law) and would lead to collapse of the alveoli if the surface tension were to remain constant. In the case of the spherical alveoli, the pressure generated by the surface tension is double that in the tubular ducts, as there are two planes of curvature. Laplace's law for a spherical shape is thus:

$$\text{Pressure gradient across the wall of a sphere} = \frac{2 \times \text{Tension}}{\text{Radius}}$$

Surfactant, present in the lining fluid of the alveoli, protects the patient from this danger by two mechanisms. It reduces the surface tension of the fluid lining the alveoli appreciably and renders the surface tension variable, so the tension increases as the alveoli distend and decreases as the alveoli contract, thus preventing collapse. In premature infants, surfactant may not yet be present in the alveoli and, consequently, problems may arise because of alveolar collapse and failure of alveoli to open. In the case of the two alveoli shown in Fig. 2.11, lack of surfactant would cause the smaller alveolus to collapse, transferring the gas to the larger one.

Viscosity

In addition to changes of vessel and airway diameters due to tension in the walls, viscosity of the contained fluid, especially if liquid, may also affect flow. In the circulation, for example, blood viscosity is increased if haemoglobin concentration is

Figure 2.11 Alveoli of different diameters

300 μm diameter

150 μm diameter

raised. A rise in viscosity reduces blood flow, giving a risk of vascular occlusion. Viscosity increases at low temperature, with patient age and with cigarette smoking, whereas treatment with low-molecular-weight dextran reduces it. The viscosity of blood is anomalous because blood is not a uniform fluid but contains cells. This leads to a rise in the viscosity of blood at very low flows such as those which occur in areas with intermittent circulation.

A viscometer is used to measure viscosity. In a typical viscometer, a sample of blood is placed in a cone-shaped cup which is maintained at a set temperature. The cup is rotated or oscillated. A cone-shaped probe within the cup is dragged by the viscosity of the blood and the torque generated is used to provide a measure of the viscosity.

Other viscometers determine viscosity by measuring the time taken for a sample of liquid to flow down a vertical tube. The transit time is measured by detecting the meniscus position with photocells and the viscosity can then be computed electronically from this transit time.

Flow through a Venturi

Some equipment may include a tube with a constriction in which the cross section gradually decreases and then increases. This is known as a Venturi and is illustrated in Fig. 2.12. If the pressure along the tube is measured, it is found that the pressure at the narrowest point is lower than elsewhere and is often below atmospheric pressure. This fall of pressure at a constriction in a tube is named after its discoverer, Bernoulli, and is applied in several devices.

The fall in pressure at the narrowing of a tube arises in the following way. Flowing fluid contains energy in two forms: potential energy associated with its pressure and kinetic energy associated with its flow. At a constriction, B in the diagram, there is a considerable increase of fluid velocity and a great gain of kinetic energy. Such an increase of kinetic energy can only occur if there is a fall in potential energy, because the total energy present must remain constant. In consequence, a marked fall of pressure occurs at this point to a value below the pressure at either A or C. As the tube widens, the fluid velocity falls and with it the kinetic energy component, so that the potential energy and, hence, the pressure rise. The kinetic energy of the fluid can also be converted into heat energy by friction of the moving fluid with its container or surroundings. Therefore, if the system is to work efficiently, the frictional losses which cause the change in pressure between points A and C must be small, so that a negligible amount of energy is lost as heat.

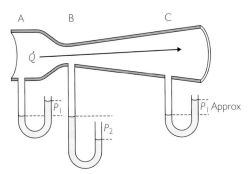

Figure 2.12 Principle of the Venturi

Consider now what happens if the pressure gauge at position P_2 is removed, leaving the side tube open. If the pressure at this point is below atmospheric pressure, air or other fluid can be entrained through the side tube. An apparatus like this is called an injector and Fig. 2.13 shows how a Venturi with an injector operates.

The driving fluid entrains fluid through a side tube because of the low pressure at the point where the fluid velocity is greatest, at the constriction. Injectors working on this principle may be used to provide suction, either water or gas being used as the driving fluid.

A nebulizer (Fig. 2.14) is another example of this principle. In this case, gas as the driving fluid enters by the centre tube, entrains liquid from a side tube and breaks it up into droplets suitable for inhalation. Nebulizers are discussed more fully in Chapter 12.

A compact source of gas for emergency use can be provided by using an injector driven with oxygen from a cylinder to entrain air. The dilution of the stored oxygen with air increases the volume of gas available.

The oxygen mask illustrated in Fig. 2.15 also makes use of an injector. There is a reduction in pressure due to the Bernoulli effect in the flow of oxygen moving at high speed after leaving the injector and this entrains air into the oxygen flow. Another factor is also present. Friction between the oxygen moving at high speed and the air pulls more air along with the flow of oxygen, an effect known as jet entrainment. This injector therefore dilutes oxygen with air and provides clinically useful concentrations. The same principle is used in other types of oxygen therapy and inhalation apparatus.

Entrainment Ratio

The total entrained flow is due both to the Bernoulli effect and jet entrainment. The entrainment ratio is defined as the ratio of entrained flow to driving flow:

Figure 2.13 Fluid entrainment by a Venturi

Figure 2.14
Principle of a
nebulizer

Water

Figure 2.15 Venturi oxygen mask

Entrained air

O_2

$$\text{Entrainment ratio} = \frac{\text{Entrained flow}}{\text{Driving flow}}$$

Thus, a 9 to 1 entrainment ratio indicates that there are 9 litres min^{-1} being entrained by a driving gas of 1 litre min^{-1}. In clinical practice, entrainment ratios may not be constant and obstruction at the outlet of the Venturi can result in a fall in the entrainment ratio. This gave rise to problems in ventilators worked by injectors in which oxygen was used to entrain air or nitrous oxide. In such cases, back pressure altered the flow and so the resulting oxygen concentration.

The Coanda Effect

As explained previously, there is a fall in pressure in fluid flowing through a tube when the tube narrows, due to the increase in speed of the stream of fluid. This low pressure can be used to entrain other fluid into the stream. If such a stream flows along a solid surface, such as the wall of a wide tube, air cannot be entrained where the stream touches the wall, so a region of low pressure remains in this area and the stream is held against the wall. Figure 2.16 illustrates this effect in a system where a narrow tube enters a Y-junction of wider bore and it is seen that, because the flow tends to cling to one side, the flow does not divide evenly between the two outlets but flows through only one limb of the 'Y'. This behaviour is known as the Coanda effect and may be of importance in explaining the uneven distribution of gas flow to alveoli where there has been a slight narrowing of the bronchiole before it divides. It may also explain some cases of myocardial infarction, where there may be narrowing before the branching of a coronary artery. In such a case, all the blood could be flowing into one limb of the coronary artery despite the fact that there is still an apparently patent lumen in the other branch.

A valve mechanism with no moving parts can be made if two tubes are inserted at each side at the exit of the narrow tube (Fig. 2.17). Flow through either of these side tubes can switch the main flow from one exit tube to the other.

Figure 2.16 Coanda effect

Area of low pressure

Figure 2.17 Valve
mechanism based on
the Coanda effect

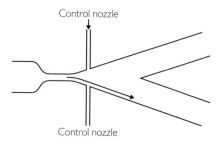

Control nozzle

Control nozzle

Having been transferred, the flow continues into the appropriate branch after the switching flow has been removed. Devices of this kind are known as fluid logic, and may be incorporated in ventilators to reduce the number of valves and moving parts. However, such ventilators consume extra gas which is used as the power for the fluid logic.

Volume and Flow Measurement

3

Volume and flow are related, for, if the volume of a fluid passing some point can be measured over a given time, the flow can be calculated. As gases are compressible, there are special problems associated with the measurement of gas flows and volumes which are not present in the case of liquids.

Gas Volume Measurement

The Benedict Roth spirometer (Fig. 3.1) was widely used for both physiological and clinical studies. A light bell moves with the patient's breathing and this movement may be recorded by a pen on a rotating drum, the motion of the bell being transferred to the pen through a connecting wire which passes over two pulleys. A water seal prevents leakage of gas from the bell and this seal is small in order to reduce the volume of gas which dissolves in the water.

An alternative system for respiratory measurements is the Vitalograph, which is more portable than the Benedict Roth spirometer.

In the Vitalograph (Fig. 3.2), bellows are used to measure gas volume. The top plate of the bellows is pivoted and its motion is transferred to a scriber which records volume changes on a chart. The chart is motor driven and automatically starts to move as soon as the bellows move from their empty position. This allows expired volume–time graphs to be plotted.

Both these spirometers are suitable for measuring limited gas volumes up to a few litres. Occasionally in anaesthesia larger volumes must be measured and in this case a dry gas meter may be used. The instrument is similar to that used in domestic gas supplies and a simplified meter is illustrated in Fig. 3.3. In this diagram two compartments are shown, A and B. In the position illustrated, gas passes into com-

Figure 3.1 Benedict Roth spirometer

Figure 3.2 Principle of the Vitalograph

Figure 3.3 Principle of action of a dry gas meter

partment B, compressing the bellows, which simultaneously empty compartment A. As the bellows are compressed, they move a lever to provide a volume recording and also move a rod CC to shift the valves to a new position (Fig. 3.4).

In this position, compartment A is now filled until it too moves the rod and lever mechanism. The system described is a simplified one and, in fact, two sets of these compartments are necessary for the meter to work continuously. There is also a set of gears to record the volume measured.

The compact Wright respirometer is more convenient for measuring tidal volumes in anaesthesia. Figure 3.5 illustrates the principle of its action. Like the dry gas meter it has a set of gears, but in this case the volume measurement is achieved by monitoring the continuous rotation of a vane as it is moved by the flow of gas. The effect of the slits is to cause a circular motion of the airflow which rotates the vane. The vane does not rotate when the flow is reversed. The Wright respirometer is calibrated for use for tidal volume measurement and for tidal ventilation. Its calibration is inaccurate if it is used to measure a continuous flow.

A disadvantage of the Wright respirometer is that it does not give an electrical output for analysis and recording, but volume monitors are available with this

Figure 3.4 Dry gas meter after movement of rod CC

Figure 3.5 Wright respirometer

facility. Figure 3.6 illustrates the principle of one type. Like the Wright respirometer, the monitor depends upon the movement of a vane mounted on jewelled bearings within the airflow. To create a spiral movement of the air in this case, the air passes through two sets of six fixed and angled blades at either side of the moving vane. The vane moves alternately clockwise and anticlockwise as the patient breathes in and out and the vane's movement is monitored by means of two infrared beams as shown. An electronic processor analyses the signal to indicate tidal volume and minute volume.

This instrument gives more accurate measurements than the mechanical Wright respirometer because the drag of the gears on the vane is eliminated, but it requires a source of electrical power and is less portable and more expensive than the simpler instrument.

In clinical practice, gas volume measurements made with the instruments described above are often at ambient temperature and pressure. For scientific and research work, however, volumes are corrected to a standard temperature and pressure (STP), as described in Chapter 4.

Figure 3.6 Electronic volume monitor

Liquid Volume Measurement

Liquid volume measurement can often be made simply by collecting the volume in a measuring cylinder. For measurement of blood volume in the body more advanced techniques are required, such as those which use the dilution of an indicator, but it is necessary to estimate both the red cell and plasma volumes.

Dilution Techniques

For red cell volume measurement, red cells which have been specially identified by radioactive labelling are used (Chapter 24). Suppose a known amount or dose of these labelled red cells is injected into a patient. After they have mixed thoroughly with the patient's blood, the concentration of the labelled cells may be deduced from the radioactivity of a blood sample from the patient:

$$\text{Concentration of labelled red cells} = \frac{\text{Dose of labelled red cells}}{\text{Red cell volume}}$$

Therefore:

$$\text{Red cell volume} = \frac{\text{Dose of labelled red cells}}{\text{Concentration of labelled red cells}}$$

For measuring plasma volume, the same dilution technique is used with radioactive albumin instead of radioactive labelled red cells. The total blood volume can then be calculated by adding together the plasma and red cell volumes. It is possible to estimate blood volume from either of these determinations provided that the ratio of red cell volume to blood volume is known from a haematocrit reading:

$$\text{Blood volume} = \frac{\text{Red cell volume}}{\text{Haematocrit}}$$

$$\text{Blood volume} = \frac{\text{Plasma volume}}{1 - \text{Haematocrit}}$$

Clinically, these dilution techniques have limitations, because in shocked patients, pooling and stasis of blood may occur in poorly perfused areas and even mixing of the radioactive indicator may not be obtained. In cases of polycythaemia, the blood sample haematocrit might be different from the whole body haematocrit, so both red cell volume and plasma volume would need to be measured in order to estimate blood volume.

A similar dilution technique employing radioactive sodium has been used to measure total extracellular volume.

Gas Flow Measurement

Anaesthetists require a continuous indication of gas flows in the anaesthetic machine and this is provided by a variable orifice flowmeter, often referred to by the trade name of Rotameter. Figure 3.7A illustrates the flowmeter. A bobbin is supported in the middle of a tapered glass or plastic tube by the gas flow and, as the flow increases, the bobbin rises in the tube and the clearance round the bobbin increases. In other words, there is a variable orifice round the bobbin which depends on the gas flow. The pressure across the bobbin remains constant because it gives rise to a force which balances the force of gravity on the bobbin. The

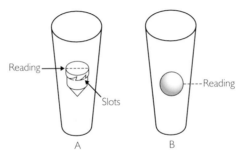

Reading

Slots

Reading

A   B

Figure 3.7 Variable orifice flowmeters

increase in the area of the annular orifice as the bobbin rises reduces flow resistance at higher flows and so the pressure across the bobbin stays constant, despite the flow increase.

Small slots are placed round the top of the bobbin as shown, causing it to rotate centrally in the gas flow. In this type of flowmeter, readings are made from the upper surface of the bobbin.

In a variable orifice flowmeter, there is a mixture of turbulent and laminar flow, and so for calibration purposes both the density and viscosity of the fluid are important (Chapter 2). Consequently, careful recalibration is required if a flowmeter is used for a different fluid than that for which it was initially designed.

The flowmeter tube must be kept vertical to obtain a correct reading and to prevent the bobbin touching the sides of the tube and sticking. Sticking is more likely to occur when the bobbin is rotating near the bottom of the tube. Electrostatic charges may also build up on the bobbin if it rubs against the side of the tube, and these may increase the tendency to stick. To prevent the build-up of such charges, some tubes have a conductive strip running down the inside at the back, whereas in others a clear conductive coating is provided inside to conduct away any electrostatic charges.

The problem of sticking is less if a simple ball flowmeter is used as shown in Fig. 3.7B, but this may be less accurate because there is no well-defined surface to read. In practice, the readings are taken from the middle of the ball.

In the illustration (Fig. 3.7), the flowmeters have a bore with a simple straight wall taper but in practice the bore is usually specially moulded with a varying taper so that both low and high flows can be measured conveniently. This is essential if anaesthetists wish to use the same flowmeter for low flows to a closed circuit and also for high-flow systems. Added accuracy can be achieved if two flowmeters, one for low and one for high flows, are used in series. With such systems, newer flowmeters normally indicate flows within 2.5% of the true value, whereas inaccuracies of over 5% have been reported with older types of flowmeter.

Below the flowmeter, there is usually a needle valve, as illustrated in Fig. 3.8. In the needle valve there is a spindle, attached to a control knob which screws into the seating of the inlet to turn off the gas supply to the flowmeter above. Leakage of gas around the spindle is prevented by a gland with its gland nut. A gland is a washer of compressible material, and glands and gland nuts are also used to prevent leakage on gas cylinders. At the bottom of each flowmeter, a dust filter of sintered metal is also present.

The principle of flow through the valve differs from that described in Chapter 2 in that, at a normal gas supply pressure, the linear velocity of the gas round the

Figure 3.8 Needle valve

control spindle approaches the speed of sound and achieves a constant maximum value. Consequently, the flow only depends upon the area of the channel and is unaffected by small changes of upstream pressure, e.g. at the outlet of the flowmeters. This is an advantage to the anaesthetist as it means that the gas flows, once set, do not alter when additional apparatus such as a vaporizer or lung ventilator is attached at the outlet of the flowmeters, though the bobbin position may alter slightly, as described later.

The positions of individual gas flowmeters on the anaesthetic machine may cause problems, as illustrated in Fig. 3.9A. If there is a leak in the centre flowmeter or in the centre of the block, more oxygen (from the left) leaks out through this hole than nitrous oxide, resulting in a higher percentage of nitrous oxide than intended being delivered to the patient, perhaps with fatal consequences.

One solution would be to reverse the oxygen and nitrous oxide flowmeter positions, as shown in Fig. 3.9B; these positions may be found in North America. Unfortunately, many anaesthetists are so used to the current position that this solution is not universally acceptable. Therefore, on some machines another solution, illustrated in Fig. 3.9C, is found. Here there is suitable channelling present in order to pick up the oxygen selectively.

As an additional safety measure it is now recommended that there should be no risk of administration of less than 25% oxygen. One mechanism used to

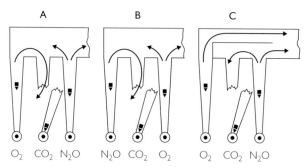

Figure 3.9 The risk of hypoxia with a faulty flowmeter block and possible design measures to prevent it

achieve this is a chain linking the oxygen and nitrous oxide flowmeter controls. With this system, opening the nitrous oxide flowmeter valve also rotates the oxygen control and opens the oxygen valve, so oxygen always flows when nitrous oxide is turned on. Pneumatic mixing valves have also been used to give the same effect.

From the outlets of the flowmeters, the gas may pass through a vaporizer and a ventilator and the additional resistance to gas flow through these machines may cause the pressure to increase at the outlet of the flowmeters. A pressure increase affects calibration due to alteration in the density and viscosity of the gases. There is then a slight inaccuracy in the indicated flow, even if a correction is made for the re-expansion of gas to ambient pressure. Some flowmeters now have the flow controls on the outlet so that they are pressurized and calibrated to work at an increased pressure of several bar, which minimizes the effect of the relatively smaller pressure changes at the outlet.

A second instrument which measures flow by the variable orifice principle is the Wright peak flowmeter illustrated in Fig. 3.10. In this flowmeter the patient's expired gases are directed against a movable vane causing it to rotate. As the vane rotates, it opens up a circular slot around the base of the instrument and so allows the gases to escape.

Rotation of the vane is opposed by the force from a coiled spring and a pointer mounted on the axis of the vane registers its movement on a calibrated dial. The spring force is relatively constant and its action on the area of the vane gives a very small steady pressure to balance the constant pressure driving the flow of gas through the variable orifice. The size of this orifice increases to that required for the gas flow and, at peak flow, the vane reaches a maximum position from which it is prevented from returning by a ratchet. After the maximum reading is taken, the vane can be released by depressing a button and the pointer returns to zero. An alternative, more compact, peak flowmeter has a cylindrical shape and the air escapes from a straight slot in place of the circular one described. However, the variable orifice principle is still used. For an adult a peak flow of 400–500 litres min^{-1} is common, but in a patient with emphysema this may be below 100 litres min^{-1}.

A common technique for obtaining an electrical signal proportional to flow is the use of the pneumotachograph (Fig. 3.11). The flow-measuring unit of this instrument contains a gauze screen which has a sufficiently large diameter to ensure laminar flow through the gauze. The gauze acts as a resistance to flow, so

Figure 3.10 Wright peak flowmeter

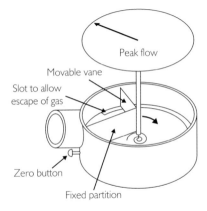

Peak flow

Movable vane

Slot to allow escape of gas

Zero button

Fixed partition

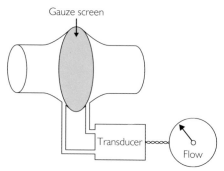

Figure 3.11 Pneumotachograph

respiratory airflow from the patient causes a small pressure drop across the gauze. This pressure change is measured by a transducer, which converts the pressure change into an electrical signal, which in turn can be displayed and recorded. (The word transducer describes a device which changes a signal from one form of energy to another.)

The pneumotachograph can measure rapid changes in the patient's respiration, at the same time avoiding any appreciable resistance to breathing. As laminar flow depends on fluid viscosity, changes in the composition or temperature of the gas passing through the pneumotachograph affect its accuracy; the addition of anaesthetic gases, for example, can affect the calibration. To overcome the problem of inaccuracy due to variation in gas temperature, some pneumotachographs are maintained at a constant temperature by a heating element. This also has the advantage of preventing water vapour in the expired gas from condensing out on the gauze. In addition to its use to measure flow, the pneumotachograph may be used to record volume by integrating the flow through it electronically.

An alternative form of the pneumotachograph, shown in Fig. 3.12, uses tubes aligned with the direction of fluid flow, which are known as Pitot tubes.

The Pitot tubes are connected to a differential pressure transducer. Thus, fluid in each of the Pitot tubes is stationary, although fluid in the section of the breathing system in which they are located may be moving. The pressure in the tube which faces into the direction of fluid flow is greater than the pressure that is present when the fluid is not moving. The kinetic energy of the moving fluid is converted to potential energy in the tube, which results in an increase of pressure in the tube. Kinetic energy is proportional to the square of fluid velocity and potential energy is proportional to pressure. The pressure measured by the Pitot tube that faces into the direction of fluid flow is proportional to the kinetic energy and therefore to the square of the fluid velocity. The velocity of the fluid flow varies

Figure 3.12 Measurement of flow with Pitot tubes

Figure 3.13 Principle of the electronic mass flowmeter

across the diameter of the breathing system, but the Pitot tubes can be used to measure flow through the breathing system provided that the velocity measured at the one point across the diameter by the Pitot tubes remains proportional to the total flow through the breathing system as the flow varies. The breathing system adaptor in which the Pitot tubes are located is designed to achieve this, so that flow is related to velocity.

Another device giving an electronic output is the mass flowmeter, the principle of one form of which is illustrated in Fig. 3.13. Electric current passes through a thermistor, an electronic component, the resistance of which varies with temperature. The current heats the thermistor and the gas flow being measured passes the thermistor, carrying away heat energy. To maintain the thermistor at a constant temperature, the electric current must be increased if the gas flow increases, since an increased gas flow carries away more heat energy. Thus, the current required is a measure of the gas flow.

The measurement process is also affected by the temperature of the gas flow, since cool gas removes more heat from the thermistor than warm gas. Compensation for this effect is applied by measuring the temperature of the gas flow with a second thermistor before the flow has passed over the thermistor used for flow measurement.

Liquid Flow Measurement

The measurement of intravenous fluid infusion rate is perhaps the most common type of liquid flow measurement in anaesthesia, as the drops passing through the drip chamber of a fluid or blood administration set provide a quick visual indication of flow. In addition, these drops have a nominal volume which permits a measure of the infusion rate to be made. This is obtained by multiplying the drop volume by the rate at which the drops pass through the chamber.

Surface tension is one of the factors determining the final diameter of a drop forming at the end of a tube through which liquid is flowing slowly. As the drop forms, the surface tension on its surface balances the force of gravity on the liquid in the drop and prevents the drop detaching from the end of the tube. As the size increases, the weight of the drop eventually becomes too large to be supported by the surface tension and the drop detaches from the end of the tube. The final volume of the drop depends on the density and surface tension of the liquid, the size and shape of the tube, and the rate at which liquid is flowing through the tube. Density and surface tension depend in turn on the temperature and nature of the solution or of the blood being transfused, so that variations of 20% of the nominal drop volume, and hence of the estimated flow, are possible.

Infusion controllers and pumps are available which determine the infusion rate by counting drops passing through a drip chamber. However, these should not be relied upon to control an infusion with complete accuracy. Infusion sets are available with different calibrations expressed in drops per millilitre, and care should be taken to use the correct set for a particular pump.

The drip counter of an infusion controller is shown clipped onto the drip chamber of an infusion set in Fig. 3.14.

A beam of light or infrared radiation, produced by a lamp or light-emitting diode, passes through the chamber to strike a photodetector on the other side. The light intensity falling on the photodetector is reduced every time a drop interrupts the beam. Thus, the controller is able to count the drip rate and adjust the flow of liquid to some set value. This adjustment is carried out automatically by the pressure of a bar against a length of delivery tubing clamped in the controller. Movement of the bar flattens the tubing, increasing the resistance to flow and decreasing the rate of infusion.

For reliable operation, drip counters should be positioned carefully so that the light beam is halfway between the drop-forming orifice and the liquid level. The liquid should occupy one-third of the drip chamber, which should be vertical so that the drops interrupt the light beam correctly.

The system described uses the force of gravity to supply the liquid to the drip chamber. Alternatively, infusion fluid may be pumped to the patient. A volumetric pump may use a disposable cassette which has one or more pistons and valves and is loaded into a motorized holder. In this instance, the volume of liquid administered and its flow can be accurately known and the problems associated with drip counters are avoided. Ordinary syringes, preloaded with a required drug, can also be used in a suitable motorized holder to infuse a small volume of fluid accurately.

Following the introduction of intravenous hypnotics such as propofol, and opioids such as alfentanil and remifentanil, special infusion pumps have been designed for use during anaesthesia. These pumps differ from the standard systems used in wards by being able to deliver much faster infusion rates, e.g. over 1000 ml h^{-1} for propofol. Some have electromagnetically encoded cards which fit on the front of the device over the setting dials and communicate the drug type and

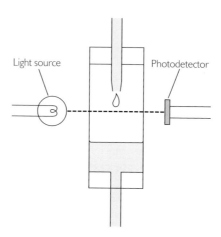

Figure 3.14 Drip counter of an infusion controller

Light source

Photodetector

concentration to the pump. The appropriate infusion rate is calculated automatically once the dose in $\mu g\ kg^{-1}\ min^{-1}$ and the patient's weight have been selected with dials on the infusion pump. Thus, the anaesthetist does not need to prescribe an infusion rate in $ml\ h^{-1}$.

The most recent types of infusion systems used for intravenous anaesthesia are called target-controlled infusion (TCI) systems. These microprocessor-based infusion devices incorporate a three-compartment pharmacokinetic model which describes the distribution and elimination of the drug. The TCI system allows the desired target blood concentration of propofol considered appropriate for any individual patient and level of surgical stimulation to be achieved and maintained at any time.

High pressures can readily be developed when syringes are used (Chapter 1), and so there is a need for particular care when positioning an intravascular cannula for use with an infusion pump.

If it is necessary to check the flow of liquid from some apparatus, then a burette or measuring cylinder and a stopwatch or timer may suffice. Variable orifice flowmeters may also be used for liquids as well as gases; for example, such flowmeters may be used to measure flow through renal dialysis or heart-lung bypass equipment. In the case of flows in the circulation, however, more advanced techniques are required and these include dye dilution, isotope dilution and thermal dilution (Chapter 5), ultrasonic measurement (Chapter 13) and the electromagnetic flowmeter (Chapter 14). In addition to these special techniques, the Fick principle is particularly important.

The Fick Principle

The example given in Fig. 3.15 illustrates the principle for the calculation of pulmonary blood flow from the oxygen uptake in the lungs. The patient rebreathes oxygen into a Benedict Roth spirometer through a soda lime absorber, and the rate of uptake of oxygen is shown by the slope of the tracing to be $250\ ml\ min^{-1}$. From a catheter in the right atrium or pulmonary artery a sample of mixed venous blood is obtained and analysed to show an oxygen content of $150\ ml\ litre^{-1}$ of blood. An arterial blood sample shows the arterial blood oxygen concentration to be $200\ ml\ litre^{-1}$. Each litre of blood therefore gains an extra $50\ ml$ of oxygen in its passage through the lungs. Since $250\ ml$ of oxygen is being taken up in the lungs each minute, $250/50$, i.e. 5 litres of blood, must flow through the lungs to carry this volume.

Figure 3.15 Fick principle

In this example, blood flow has been calculated using the oxygen uptake in the lungs. Alternatively, the Fick principle could be applied to calculate the blood flow from the pulmonary carbon dioxide excretion and carbon dioxide concentrations in arterial and mixed venous blood samples.

The Fick principle can be applied in general to measure blood flow to an organ where there is a steady flow of a substance to or from the organ, the concentration of which can be measured.

The general formula is:

Blood flow to the organ =

$$\frac{\text{Rate of uptake or excretion of a substance}}{\text{Difference in concentration of the substance in arterial and venous blood}}$$

Noninvasive Cardiac Output Measurement by Use of the Differential Fick Principle to Measure Elimination of Carbon Dioxide

This technique can be used with ventilated patients. Applying the Fick principle to the measurement of cardiac output gives the following relationship:

Cardiac output =

$$\frac{\text{Rate of elimination of carbon dioxide from the lungs } (\dot{V})}{\text{Venous concentration of carbon dioxide } (v) - \text{arterial concentration of carbon dioxide } (a)}$$

If expired gas is rebreathed, the arterial concentration of carbon dioxide rises, since this depends on the inspired concentration of carbon dioxide. Thus two versions of the above equation can be written – one that applies to normal breathing and one that applies to rebreathing:

$$\text{Cardiac output} = \frac{\dot{V}_n}{v_n - a_n} \quad \text{and Cardiac output} = \frac{\dot{V}_r}{v_r - a_r}$$

Rearranging these equations gives

$$v_n - a_n = \frac{\dot{V}_n}{\text{Cardiac output}} \quad \text{and} \quad v_r - a_r = \frac{\dot{V}_r}{\text{Cardiac output}}$$

It has been shown that mixed venous carbon dioxide concentration does not change significantly throughout a 50 s period of rebreathing, so, since $v_n = v_r$ under these circumstances

$$a_n + \frac{\dot{V}_n}{\text{Cardiac output}} = a_r + \frac{\dot{V}_r}{\text{Cardiac output}}$$

$$a_n \times \text{Cardiac output} - a_r \times \text{Cardiac output} = \dot{V}_r - \dot{V}_n$$

So

$$\text{Cardiac output} = \frac{\dot{V}_r - \dot{V}_n}{a_n - a_r}$$

This expression permits cardiac output determination from noninvasive physiological measurements. The principle of the equipment used to implement this technique is shown in Fig. 3.16.

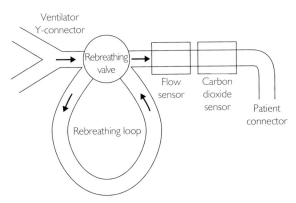

Figure 3.16 Principle of a noninvasive cardiac output measurement technique

The system containing the sensors and valve is placed between the patient connector and the ventilator Y-connector. Every 3 min, the patient's inspired and expired gases are automatically diverted through the rebreathing loop for 50 s by a rebreathing valve.

At any time, the rate of elimination of carbon dioxide from the lungs is

$\dot{V}$ = Expiratory flow × Fraction of carbon dioxide present in this expiratory flow

This product is averaged over the breathing cycle to obtain a value for use in the formula. End-tidal carbon dioxide concentration is used to estimate the arterial carbon dioxide concentration. When the Fick principle is applied as described, the resulting value for cardiac output represents only the fraction of the flow that participates in gas exchange, i.e. the pulmonary capillary blood flow. A method is therefore needed to estimate the shunt flow, so this can be added to the value obtained from the measurement. This is done by taking a value for the inspired oxygen concentration entered into the equipment by the operator and comparing the expected oxygen saturation with oxygen saturation measured by means of pulse oximetry.

The Gas Laws

4

Molecular Theory

A brief review of molecular theory is given first because it helps in understanding the gas laws.

All substances are composed of atoms or compounds of atoms, i.e. molecules. In a solid, the atoms or molecules are usually arranged in a regular formation called a lattice and each molecule in the lattice exerts forces on its neighbours and is continuously in motion, oscillating about a mean position. If heat is added to a solid, each molecule vibrates with a greater amplitude and therefore takes up a greater amount of space. The molecules move further apart and, consequently, the force exerted by each on its neighbours is reduced. Eventually the forces are not sufficient to hold the molecules together in a lattice, although smaller groupings remain. The lattice breaks down; the substance melts and turns into a liquid. In a liquid, the molecules still exert some influence on each other and the forces of attraction between them are called van der Waals forces. The molecules in a liquid have more vibrational energy than in a solid and each molecule can move about through the liquid. If heat is added to a liquid, each molecule gains further kinetic energy and eventually some molecules are able to overcome the van der Waals forces exerted by their neighbours and are able to move about in space. This state is that of a gas or vapour.

Figure 4.1 illustrates the interface between a liquid and its vapour. Molecules at the surface of the liquid occasionally escape, as shown at 'A' in the diagram. Conversely, molecules of gas moving towards the liquid may transfer into the liquid phase, as shown at 'B'. Eventually, at any one temperature an equilibrium

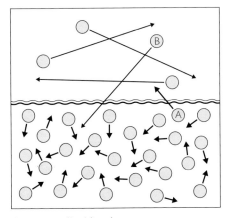

Figure 4.1 Interface between a liquid and a gas

Figure 4.2 Gas in a syringe model to illustrate molecular theory

occurs between these two rates of molecular transfer and the vapour above the liquid is said to be at its saturated vapour pressure.

If the liquid is heated to its boiling point, the energy of the molecules is so great that they all transfer to the gaseous phase. In a gas, the molecules collide with each other and with the walls of a container at frequent intervals. The result of the collisions between the molecules of a gas and the walls of the container is that a force is exerted on the walls and this force exerted over a certain area is defined as the pressure.

The Gas Laws

Figure 4.2 illustrates a volume of gas within a large syringe. The collisions between the molecules and the walls of the container result in an absolute pressure P, which in this case is a typical atmospheric pressure of 100 kPa (1 bar). If this syringe is at a constant temperature, the molecules will have a certain energy of motion and will therefore collide with the walls of the container at a given frequency.

If the temperature is kept constant and the volume of the container is reduced (Fig. 4.3), the molecules will still have the same energy of motion but, as they are in a smaller volume, they will collide with the walls of the container more frequently. The greater the number of collisions with the walls, the greater the pressure of the gas in the container. Halving the volume V of the syringe, as in Fig. 4.3, doubles the absolute pressure P from 100 to 200 kPa.

$$V \propto \frac{1}{P}$$

$$PV = \text{constant } (k_1)$$

Figure 4.3 Effect of volume change at constant temperature

Figure 4.4 Use of Boyle's law to calculate the content of an oxygen cylinder

This is the first perfect gas law, Boyle's law:

Boyle's law states that at constant temperature the volume of a given mass of gas varies inversely with the absolute pressure.

Figure 4.4 provides an example of the application of Boyle's law. On the left is shown a typical large oxygen cylinder such as is used in oxygen therapy. How much oxygen will be available at atmospheric pressure? The internal capacity of the cylinder is about 10 litres and when full it has a gauge pressure of 137 bar or 13,700 kPa. If the atmospheric pressure is 100 kPa, the total or absolute pressure of the oxygen will be 13,800 kPa, since absolute pressure is gauge pressure plus atmospheric pressure. The calculations are given on the right of the diagram and the total volume of oxygen works out at 1380 litres. As 10 litres are retained in the 'empty' oxygen cylinder, 1370 litres are available for delivery at atmospheric pressure.

Consider now a gas maintained at constant pressure (Fig. 4.5). In the example shown, this means that the barrel of the syringe is allowed to move freely to

Figure 4.5 Effect of change of temperature at constant pressure

maintain the ambient pressure of 100 kPa. If heat is added to the volume of gas, as in the lower diagram, the energy of movement of the molecules increases and this results in more collisions with the walls of the container. In order that the frequency of collisions, and thus the pressure, remains constant the volume must increase. Thus, if the absolute temperature T in the syringe is doubled from 273 K to 546 K, it is found that the volume V in the syringe also doubles.

$$V \propto T$$

$$\frac{V}{T} = \text{constant } (k_2)$$

This is the second perfect gas law, known also as Charles' law or Gay Lussac's law:

Charles' law states that at constant pressure the volume of a given mass of gas varies directly with the absolute temperature.

This law shows that gases expand when they are heated and so become less dense. It means too that warm air tends to rise and this causes convection currents, which are considered in Chapter 9.

The third of the gas laws is illustrated in Fig. 4.6, in which a syringe is maintained at constant volume. If heat is added to this constant volume container, the molecules of the gas gain kinetic energy and collide with the walls of the container more frequently, thus resulting in an increase in pressure. Consequently, at constant volume, a change in absolute temperature T in a gas produces a change in pressure P.

$$P \propto T$$

$$\frac{P}{T} = \text{constant } (k_3)$$

The third perfect gas law states that at constant volume the absolute pressure of a given mass of gas varies directly with the absolute temperature.

An application of this law is found in the hydrogen thermometer, which is used as a scientific standard for temperature measurement. When a constant volume of

Figure 4.6 Effect of change of temperature at constant volume

hydrogen is heated, the rise in pressure may be accurately recorded and it gives a measure of the absolute temperature increase.

As volumes of gases are greatly affected by changes of temperature and pressure, it is important to specify the temperature and pressure at which any measurement of volume is made. Moreover, it is often useful to correct results to a standard temperature and pressure. The standard temperature used is 273.15 K (0°C), and the standard pressure 101.325 kPa (760 mmHg). This standard temperature and pressure is known as STP.

Adiabatic Changes of State in a Gas

The three gas laws describe the behaviour of a gas when one of the three variables – pressure, temperature or volume – is constant. For these conditions to apply, heat energy is required to be added to or taken from a gas as the change occurs. The state of a gas can also be altered without allowing the gas to exchange heat energy with its surroundings, and this is called an adiabatic change. An example of such a change occurs when air is compressed in an air supply unit; the temperature of the air rises because of the compression and so a system of cooling is needed (Chapter 21). As a second example, if a gas cylinder connected to an anaesthetic machine or regulator is turned on quickly, the pressure of gas in the connecting pipes and gauges rises rapidly. Thus, the gas is compressed adiabatically and a large temperature rise, with the associated risk of fire, can occur. Alternatively, if a compressed gas expands adiabatically, cooling occurs, as in the cryoprobe.

The Cryoprobe

The cryoprobe is used for rapid freezing of tissues in the treatment of skin lesions, in gynaecology, and in ophthalmic surgery. When applied to nerves it causes local degeneration of nerve bundles and this results in long-term (3–6 months) local analgesia. This action has been used in the treatment of pain. The cooling of a cryoprobe is the result of an adiabatic process. Gas is allowed to expand rapidly out of a capillary tube and a fall in temperature occurs as a result of the expansion. The cooling effect arises from the fact that energy is required as a gas expands to overcome the van der Waals forces of attraction between the molecules of the gas. In a rapid expansion, heat exchange does not take place between the gas and its surroundings, so the energy required comes from the kinetic energy of the gas molecules themselves, which results in the gas cooling as it expands.

The elements of a typical cryoprobe are shown in Fig. 4.7. Nitrous oxide or carbon dioxide is a suitable gas and the gas flows from the cylinder through an

Figure 4.7 Principle of the cryoprobe

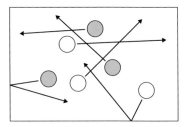

Figure 4.8 Gas mixture in a container

adjustable pressure regulator, which may be used to set the cooling rate. The gas flows through a capillary tube in the cryoprobe and expands in the probe tip, where a temperature as low as −70°C may be produced. A foot- or hand-operated valve may be used to control the flow of gas through the probe and hence the cooling effect.

Dalton's Law of Partial Pressures

Figure 4.8 illustrates a mixture of gases in a container. Pressure in the container is related to the frequency of collisions and to the mass and velocity of the molecules of the gas. In a mixture, each type of molecule contributes to the pressure exerted on the walls of the container and because each molecule behaves almost independently of its neighbours, the pressure attributable to any one type of molecule is the same whether the other type of molecule is present or not. This phenomenon was first established by John Dalton and is known as Dalton's law of partial pressures:

Dalton's law of partial pressures states that in a mixture of gases the pressure exerted by each gas is the same as that which it would exert if it alone occupied the container.

In anaesthesia the partial pressures of gases in a mixture are often of interest.

The left of Fig. 4.9 illustrates an Entonox cylinder emptied to an ambient pressure of 100 kPa. The mixture remaining in the cylinder is 50% nitrous oxide

Figure 4.9 Application of Dalton's law in an Entonox cylinder

and 50% oxygen and so each gas occupies half the cylinder volume. According to Dalton's law, the pressure exerted by the nitrous oxide in the cylinder is the same as it would exert if it alone occupied the container. But if it were to do this, the available space for the nitrous oxide would have increased from half the cylinder to a full cylinder. In other words, it would have doubled its volume. Using Boyle's law it may be calculated that the pressure in the cylinder in this case would therefore be halved from 100 kPa to 50 kPa. From these calculations it is seen that the partial pressure of this nitrous oxide is 50 kPa and, similarly, the oxygen pressure is also 50 kPa. So by applying Boyle's law and Dalton's law, the partial pressure of a gas in a mixture is obtained by multiplying the total pressure by the fractional concentration of the gas.

A second example is illustrated by Fig. 4.10, using a cylinder of air at an ambient pressure of 100 kPa. The 20.93% oxygen in the air exerts a pressure of 20.93 kPa and, ignoring the presence of other gases, the nitrogen pressure is 79.07 kPa. The calculations can also be made in terms of millimetres of mercury pressure, remembering that an ambient pressure of 100 kPa represents about 750 mmHg. The oxygen partial pressure works out at 157 mmHg, and nitrogen at 593 mmHg.

In the case of humidified gases such as those in the alveoli, the presence of water vapour must be taken into account when calculating partial pressures. Suppose, for example, a meter indicates an end-tidal carbon dioxide concentration of 5.6% measured as a dry gas. Ambient pressure is 101.3 kPa. To find the true pressure of the alveolar carbon dioxide $PACO_2$, it is not sufficient to multiply the 5.6% by the ambient pressure, as the alveolar gas is fully humidified. From an ambient pressure of 101.3 kPa, the water vapour pressure of 6.3 kPa must be subtracted before multiplying by the 5.6%:

$$PACO_2 = (101.3 - 6.3) \times \frac{5.6}{100} \text{ kPa}$$

$$= 5.3 \text{ kPa}$$

The alveolar carbon dioxide pressure is 5.3 kPa. If the calculation is made in millimetres of mercury, the alveolar carbon dioxide pressure is found to be 40 mmHg. Another example of the effect of humidity on the partial pressure of gases is given in Chapter 19.

Manufacturers make use of Dalton's law when filling cylinders with gas mixtures. Figure 4.11 illustrates the filling of a cylinder to produce a 10% carbon diox-

Figure 4.10 Application of Dalton's law in an air cylinder

Figure 4.11 Dalton's law in the filling of a cylinder of 10% carbon dioxide in oxygen

ide in oxygen mixture. The cylinder is first filled with carbon dioxide to an absolute pressure of 13.8 bar. At this pressure carbon dioxide is still gaseous at room temperature. Oxygen is then added to a total absolute pressure of 138 bar. The overall percentage of carbon dioxide is then 10%, the same as the ratio of the pressures.

Avogadro's Hypothesis

Consider the situation illustrated in Fig. 4.12. Two syringes, each of volume V, are shown containing two different gases, oxygen and hydrogen, maintained at the same temperature. If the appropriate gas molecules are added to each until the pressures in the two syringes are the same, it is found that each syringe must contain the same number of molecules. The fact that there are equal numbers of molecules is known as Avogadro's hypothesis:

Avogadro's hypothesis states that equal volumes of gases at the same temperature and pressure contain equal numbers of molecules.

Note that, as the molecular weights of oxygen and hydrogen are different, the masses of the gases in the syringes must be different. Thus, rather than express a

Figure 4.12 Syringes of gas at the same volume, pressure and temperature contain the same number of molecules

One mole of atoms of carbon 12

Figure 4.13 The mole

quantity of gas in terms of mass, it is more convenient to use a concept related to the number of molecules. This is the mole (Fig. 4.13).

A mole is the quantity of a substance containing the same number of particles as there are atoms in 0.012 kg of carbon 12. This number of particles is 6.022×10^{23} and is known as Avogadro's number. One mole of any gas at STP occupies 22.4 litres, so 2 g of hydrogen or 32 g of oxygen or 44 g of carbon dioxide occupy 22.4 litres at STP.

As an example of the mole and Avogadro's hypothesis, consider the technique of calibration of a vaporizer illustrated in Fig. 4.14. For convenience, measurements are given as at STP. On the left of the figure a steady stream of oxygen is shown flowing into the vaporizer and completely vaporizing the 18.45 g of isoflurane into a volume of 224 litres. The molecular weight of isoflurane is 184.5, so 184.5 g of isoflurane is equal to 1 mol and would occupy 22.4 litres at STP. The 18.45 g in the vaporizer is equal to 0.1 mol and would occupy 0.1×22.4 litres or 2.24 litres. This isoflurane, however, has been vaporized into a volume of 224 litres and therefore the concentration of isoflurane is 2.24/224 or 1%.

If measurements were made at temperatures and pressures other than STP, the appropriate gas laws would need to be applied and suitable corrections made. A small error may be introduced because isoflurane vapour does not obey the gas laws as closely as a gas such as hydrogen, but the results still provide a good approximation.

A similar example is illustrated in Fig. 4.15. A typical full nitrous oxide cylinder contains 3.4 kg of nitrous oxide. The molecular weight of nitrous oxide is 44, so 1 mole is 44 g. If the measurements are made at STP, what volume of nitrous oxide is obtained from this cylinder? The calculation is as follows:

44 g (1 mol) of nitrous oxide occupies 22.4 litres at STP

Therefore:

$$3400 \text{ g of nitrous oxide occupies } 22.4 \times \frac{3,400}{44} \text{ litres} = 1730 \text{ litres}$$

Oxygen →

224 l
Oxygen/isoflurane mixture

Isoflurane
18.45 g

Figure 4.14 Calibration of a vaporizer by the use of Avogadro's hypothesis

Figure 4.15 Calculation of the volume of nitrous oxide gas available from a cylinder

The volume of nitrous oxide at STP is 1730 litres, which is about 1800 litres at 15°C.

In practice, the weight of nitrous oxide is used to indicate how full cylinders are. The weight of an empty nitrous oxide cylinder is known as the tare weight and is stamped at the top. Consequently, by weighing the cylinder the nitrous oxide content may be calculated.

Universal Gas Constant

The concept of perfect gas laws can be combined with that of Avogadro's hypothesis and the mole as follows:

$$PV = k_1 \quad \frac{V}{T} = k_2 \quad \frac{P}{T} = k_3$$

Therefore:

$$\frac{PV}{T} = \text{constant}$$

It is found that PV/T equals a constant for a given quantity of gas and for 1 mole of any gas PV/T equals a unique constant known as the universal gas constant, R. The more generally applicable equation with slight rearrangement can be written as $PV = nRT$, where n is the number of moles of the gas.

This formula is applied in anaesthetic practice in the use of a contents gauge for a gas cylinder. The gas cylinder has a fixed volume, therefore, V in the equation is constant. R is a constant, and if the cylinder is at a fixed temperature, T is constant. Thus, from the formula, P is directly proportional to n, the number of moles. The pressure in the cylinder is therefore directly proportional to the number of moles in the cylinder and so to the amount of gas in the cylinder. The pressure gauge thus acts as a contents gauge provided the cylinder contains a gas.

Critical Temperature

It has been assumed that all gases obey the gas laws perfectly, but in practice slight deviations occur. Hydrogen obeys the gas laws most closely and for this reason the hydrogen thermometer is used for measurements in the international temperature scale. As the temperature of a gas approaches its boiling point, the behaviour of the gas deviates from the gas laws.

Figure 4.16 compares the filling of a nitrous oxide cylinder with that of an oxygen cylinder at an ambient temperature of 20°C. In the top diagram, nitrous oxide is being pumped under pressure into the cylinder but, once a certain pressure has been reached, the nitrous oxide liquefies without further increase of

Figure 4.16 Filling of nitrous oxide and oxygen cylinders

pressure until the cylinder is filled to the appropriate level. This contrasts with oxygen, for which, as it is pumped into the cylinder, the pressure gauge indicates accurately how full the cylinder is. No matter how much pressure is applied to the cylinder it is impossible to turn the oxygen into its liquid form at normal room temperature. If, instead, the oxygen cylinder were filled at a very low temperature, below −119°C, then it would be possible to liquefy the oxygen. In other words, it is found that there is a critical temperature for oxygen of −119°C above which oxygen cannot be liquefied by pressure alone. At or below this temperature, liquefaction under pressure is possible. Each gas has its own critical temperature.

Critical temperature is defined as the temperature above which a substance cannot be liquefied however much pressure is applied.

The critical pressure is the vapour pressure of the substance at its critical temperature. The critical temperature of nitrous oxide is 36.5°C. Consequently, the nitrous oxide in a cylinder is a gas if the temperature is above 36.5°C, as might occur in the tropics.

Figure 4.17 illustrates a large syringe of nitrous oxide at constant temperature T°C, which is above 36.5°C, and shows graphically the results of compression of the syringe. The line on the graph traces the pressure increase produced as the volume is reduced.

Figure 4.17 Pressure as a function of volume for a constant quantity of nitrous oxide at a constant temperature greater than the critical temperature

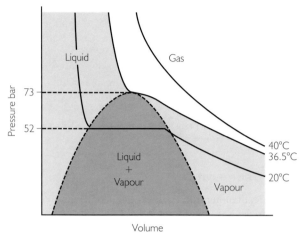

Figure 4.18 Isotherms for nitrous oxide

A series of such lines of pressure against volume can be produced at various temperatures and these are known as isotherms.

Figure 4.18 shows the isotherms for nitrous oxide at 40°C, 36.5°C and 20°C. The top line indicates the changes at 40°C. As the volume is reduced, moving from right to left on the graph, there is a smooth increase in pressure according to Boyle's law. The curve produced is a rectangular hyperbola. At the critical temperature (36.5°C), there is a critical pressure of 73 bar at which the nitrous oxide liquefies. One characteristic of a liquid is its relative incompressibility, so when the gas has completely turned to liquid, the slightest decrease in volume is associated with a great increase in pressure. An almost vertical line occurs at this point, as shown on the graph. Of greater interest is the bottom isotherm, illustrating the results at a room temperature of 20°C. As the nitrous oxide in the syringe is steadily compressed, at a pressure of 52 bar some of it liquefies, as shown in the lower area of the graph. At this point, both liquid and vapour are present and any further decrease in volume causes more vapour to condense and the pressure to remain unaltered. Consequently, a horizontal line is present on the graph at 52 bar, and this is the typical pressure in a nitrous oxide cylinder at room temperature, being its saturated vapour pressure. When all the nitrous oxide vapour is condensed into liquid, then any attempt to reduce the volume results in the sharp increase of pressure indicated by the near vertical line in this area of the graph. Note that the word nitrous oxide gas is used for the upper tracing and nitrous oxide vapour for the lower tracing. Strictly speaking the word 'gas' applies to a substance above its critical temperature, whereas 'vapour' is the word used for a substance below its critical temperature. So at normal room temperature, oxygen and nitrogen are gases, whereas nitrous oxide, carbon dioxide and isoflurane are vapours.

Consider the hypothetical case of a nitrous oxide cylinder filled completely with liquid nitrous oxide. Any increase in temperature causes the nitrous oxide to expand but, unlike a gas, a liquid is not compressible. As a result, there would be a great increase of pressure and a considerable risk of explosion. To remove this risk, the manufacturers always ensure that the cylinders are only partially filled in order to leave a volume of nitrous oxide vapour above the liquid. Any increase in temperature then causes the liquid to expand, which compresses this vapour and, as the vapour is compressed, some of it condenses, thereby keeping the pressure from rising excessively. In practice, nitrous oxide cylinders are filled according to their weight and, for a given size of cylinder, a fixed quantity of nitrous oxide is added such that space for expansion is always present in the cylinder.

The term 'filling ratio' is used to describe how much gas is used to fill a cylinder. The filling ratio is the mass of gas in a cylinder divided by the mass of water which would fill the cylinder. As 1 litre of water weighs 1 kg, the filling ratio represents the mass of nitrous oxide in kilograms divided by the internal volume of the cylinder in litres. For nitrous oxide this ratio is 0.65 in the United Kingdom.

Pseudocritical Temperature

The term 'critical temperature' applies to a single gas. When a mixture of gases is present such as the Entonox mixture of 50% nitrous oxide and 50% oxygen, there is a specific critical temperature at which the gas mixture may separate out into its constituents. This is a different concept to the critical temperature of a single gas, so the term 'pseudocritical temperature' is often used for such gas mixtures. In the case of Entonox cylinders it is found that there is a risk of separation if the temperature in the cylinder falls below −5.5°C. Such separation is most likely if the cylinder pressure before cooling is 117 bar and is found to be less likely at higher or lower pressures. In Entonox in pipelines, for instance, the pseudocritical temperature is much lower. It is below −30°C at the pipeline pressure of 4.1 bar. Consequently, there is normally no risk of separation of the nitrous oxide mixture in pipelines.

However, if cylinders are used outside in cold conditions – for example, during mountain rescue operations – it may not be possible to prevent the temperature of the cylinder contents falling to a value sufficiently low for a liquid phase to form.

Natural Exponential Functions

5

The Concept of an Exponential Process

A natural exponential function is a special form of nonlinear change often encountered in medicine and, for convenience, usually referred to as an exponential. To simplify the understanding of such a process, the filling and emptying of a bath will be used as an example. Consider first the filling of a bath with vertical sides, as shown in Fig. 5.1.

The height of the water gives a measure of the volume in the bath at any time. A graph of volume against time is linear, as would be expected from the constant flow into the bath.

Figure 5.2 shows the graph describing the emptying of the bath. Initially, emptying is fast because of the high head of water and the high pressure, but as the head of water gets less, the rate at which the bath empties becomes slower. Therefore, a plot of volume against time is a curve, steep initially and gradually getting less steep as the emptying slows, so that in theory the volume never reaches zero. This simple illustration assumes that the water in the reservoir into which the bath is emptying is at the same level as the plug hole in the bath. The water in a bath at home would normally be subject to an additional pressure head.

The process may now be analysed in greater detail. If the flow from the bath is assumed to be laminar, then the rate of flow $\dot{V}$ is directly proportional to the pressure head:

$$\dot{V} \propto P$$

Figure 5.1 The filling of a bath; a constant flow gives a linear relationship of volume V to time t

Figure 5.2 The emptying of a bath; a plot of V against t gives a curve

On the other hand, P, the pressure head of water driving the flow out, is directly proportional to V, the volume of water in the bath:

$$P \propto V$$

This arises because the bath has vertical sides, so that the height of the water surface above the bottom of the bath is a measure of its volume. The result is that the rate at which the bath empties is proportional to the volume of water in it:

$$\dot{V} \propto V$$

It is the fact that the rate at which the bath empties is proportional to the volume of water in it which makes the process exponential. At any time, the rate of change of the volume is proportional to the volume and this is an example of the definition of an exponential process:

In an exponential process the rate of change of a quantity at any time is proportional to the quantity at that time.

Figure 5.3 gives an example which is more relevant to anaesthetic practice, in which a patient is being ventilated by a constant-flow ventilator. The rate of filling of the lungs is constant, so that a graph of inspired volume against time is linear in the same way that the filling of the bath gives a linear relationship.

Figure 5.4 illustrates expiration. There is a direct analogy to the emptying of the bath and the calculations are similar. The rate of emptying is fast initially as the elastic tissues of the lungs have been stretched during inspiration, but the rate of emptying slows down as the lungs deflate. If quiet respiration is assumed, expiratory flow is predominantly laminar and is proportional to the pressure gradient P:

Since

$$\text{Laminar flow resistance} = \frac{P}{\dot{V}}$$

$$\dot{V} \propto P$$

Figure 5.3 Plot of volume as a function of time for inspiration of a patient on a constant-flow ventilator

Figure 5.4 Plot of volume as a function of time for expiration

The pressure difference P in turn is proportional to the volume of the lungs V, if it is accepted that the lungs and chest wall have a constant compliance and if V is defined as the volume of air in the lungs in excess of the functional residual capacity.

Since

$$\text{Compliance} = \frac{V}{P}$$

$$P \propto V$$

Therefore

$$\dot{V} \propto V$$

As a result, there is a direct relationship between the rate of emptying of the lungs and the volume of air in them; so the process is exponential.

Washout Curves

The graphs of such exponential processes are sometimes known as washout curves, and may describe the way in which drugs or anaesthetics are washed out of the tissues by the blood flow. To analyse this process in greater detail, another bath is considered in which the water is contaminated by a muddiness which must be washed out (Fig. 5.5). Cleaning out the muddiness could be done by running water in from the tap and running water out of the bath simultaneously at the same flow rate. Again, a simple assumption is necessary: the muddiness must remain uniformly distributed in the bath water as the water flows in and out of the bath.

In Fig. 5.5, a graph of the concentration of mud with time shows an exponential curve. Initially, when the concentration of mud is high, the mud is washed out at a high rate. Then, as the degree of muddiness decreases, the mud is washed out at a slower rate.

The rate at which the mud is removed is the flow of water through the bath multiplied by the concentration of mud in this water:

$$\dot{Q} = \dot{V} \times \text{Concentration of mud}$$

where Q is the mass of mud present in the bath, $\dot{Q}$ is the rate of removal of Q, and $\dot{V}$ is the rate of flow of water into or out of the bath.

But $\dot{V}$ is constant, therefore:

$$\dot{Q} \propto \text{Concentration of mud}$$

Figure 5.5 Plot of the concentration of mud in a bath as a function of time during the washout of mud from the bath

The actual amount of mud Q in the water at any time, however, is proportional to its concentration, as the bath has a constant volume of water in it:

$Q \propto$ Concentration of mud

Therefore:

$\dot{Q} \propto Q$

The process is exponential, as the rate of change of the quantity is proportional to the quantity present at any time.

Washout of this type occurs when indocyanine green is used to measure cardiac output (Fig. 5.6). A known amount of green indicator dye is injected via a catheter into the right heart. Using the analogy of the previous example, the bath could represent the cardiac cavities and pulmonary circulation and these contain a high concentration of green dye which is steadily washed out by the cardiac output. To sample the dye concentration from the outlet, the concentration of green dye is measured in a peripheral artery using a spectrophotometric technique. If the concentration of dye is plotted against time, a curve is obtained, as on the right of Fig. 5.6. The initial downstroke of the curve is exponential, but there is an extra hump on the right, owing to the recirculation of the dye.

If the cardiac output is high, the washout is much faster, as shown on the left of Fig. 5.7; but if the cardiac output is low, the washout of the dye is much slower, as illustrated on the right of this figure. Recirculation complicates the analysis of the curves, but one technique to overcome this difficulty includes the use of

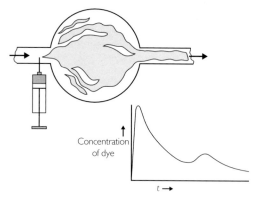

Figure 5.6 Use of a washout curve to measure cardiac output

Figure 5.7 Washout curves for a high (left) and low (right) cardiac output

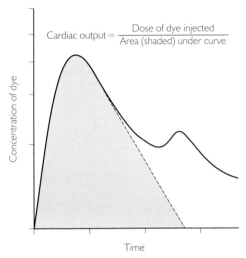

$$\text{Cardiac output} = \frac{\text{Dose of dye injected}}{\text{Area (shaded) under curve}}$$

Figure 5.8 Plot of a washout curve on semilogarithmic graph paper

semilogarithmic paper. This is graph paper on which the vertical scale is logarithmic and the horizontal scale linear (Chapter 25).

If the exponential indicator dilution curve is plotted on semilog paper, the initial downstroke is found to be a straight line (Fig. 5.8). This straight line can be prolonged downwards, thereby enclosing the stippled area shown in the figure. The cardiac output is the amount of dye injected divided by this area and the extension of this area down to a dye concentration of zero, which is not shown in its entirety in the figure since the logarithmic y axis does not extend to zero. A microprocessor is employed to make the calculations and give a readout of cardiac output.

Thermal dilution techniques are usually used to measure cardiac output in preference to the dye dilution technique.

The thermal dilution technique is shown in Fig. 5.9. A pulmonary artery catheter containing two channels is inserted into the right heart through the internal jugular vein. The distal end of the channel used for injection is inserted to the junction of the superior vena cava and right atrium. The other channel has a thermistor at its end and is guided through the right heart into the pulmonary artery. Thermistors are temperature-sensitive devices (discussed in Chapter 9). A volume of 5% dextrose, typically 10 ml in an adult, at approximately 0°C is injected through the injecting catheter. As it mixes with the warm blood in the right heart, the blood cools down and the temperature of this blood is measured as it passes over the thermistor in the pulmonary artery. A plot of temperature against time gives a washout curve as shown on the right of Fig. 5.9 and the cardiac output can be calculated from this curve in a similar manner to the dye dilution technique. The temperature scale in the illustration is inverted to show the similarity to the other washout curves. With the thermal dilution technique, however, recirculation is less evident and there is a further advantage in that repeat measurements are easier.

Another example of a washout curve – the nitrogen washout curve – occurs in one of the pulmonary function tests. In this case the patient breathes oxygen through a non-rebreathing valve, and the expired gas is analysed.

Figure 5.9 Thermal dilution technique for the measurement of cardiac output

As shown in Fig. 5.10 there is a steady decrease in the nitrogen in the lungs as it is washed out during the oxygen breathing. Normally the end-expiratory nitrogen concentration should decrease to a value below 2.5% after 7 min. Failure to do so may indicate uneven distribution of gas in the lungs.

Radioactive decay (Chapter 24) is another example of an exponential change. The rate of decay of a radioactive isotope is proportional to the quantity of isotope remaining, so it is easy to understand why the process is exponential.

Duration of Exponential Process

In all the examples of exponential processes considered so far, the quantity concerned has been diminishing and these are known as negative exponential functions. Although the quantity is decreasing, it never actually reaches zero. Consequently, the total length of time taken by the exponential process is infinite and the total time cannot be used to measure the duration of the process. Two alternative values are used instead: the half-life and the time constant.

The half-life is illustrated in Fig. 5.11. The half-life is the time taken for the quantity Q to decrease to half its initial value. After two half-lives, the quantity would of course have decreased to half of one-half, i.e. one-quarter, of the initial value and to one-eighth after three half-lives, and so on.

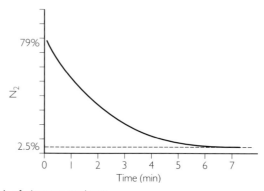

Figure 5.10 Graph of nitrogen washout

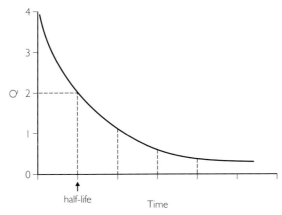

Figure 5.11 Concept of the half-life

Half-lives are often used to describe the properties of radioactive isotopes. If an isotope has a half-life of 1 hour, then after 1 hour the radioactivity is 50% of its initial value, after 2 hours 25%, after 3 hours 12.5%, and so on.

As an alternative to the half-life, the rate of an exponential process may be measured by its time constant:

The time constant is the time at which the process would have been complete had the initial rate of change continued.

The time constant is often represented by the Greek letter tau (τ), as indicated in Fig. 5.12, and is used because it results from the mathematical solution of equations used to analyse exponential processes. After 1 time constant, the quantity Q has decreased to 37% of its value: the figure of 37% arising, as mentioned above, for mathematical reasons. Consequently, the time constant is longer than the half-life. The relationship between the two is given by the expression:

half-life = time constant $\times \log_e 2$ = time constant $\times$ 0.693

To help understand the time constant, consider a definite example such as expiration. In this case a typical time constant might be 0.3 s, so after 0.3 s (1 time constant) only 37% of the tidal volume is left to be expired, after 0.6 s (2 time

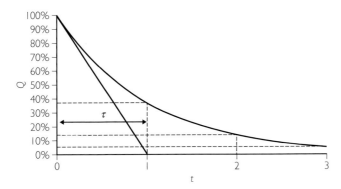

Figure 5.12 Concept of the time constant

constants) 13.5% is left, and after 0.9 s, only 5% of the tidal volume is left to be expired. Thus, expiration is 95% complete after 3 time constants.

In a normal person, almost all the tidal volume has been expired after about 1 s, so there will be little advantage in prolonging the expiratory period beyond this length of time. In the case of expiration, the time constant can be calculated if the compliance C and resistance R of the lung are known. It is obtained by the product of the two factors:

$$\tau = C \times R$$

If the lung compliance of an anaesthetized patient is 0.5 litre kPa^{-1} and the airway resistance is 0.6 kPa s litre^{-1}, then the product is 0.3 s, the figure given above as an example of an expiratory time constant.

For even distribution of the ventilation in the lungs, it is important that different parts of the lungs have the same time constant, rather than a similar resistance or a similar compliance.

Time constants have practical importance for a patient on a ventilator, as the settings for inspiratory and expiratory times are determined to some extent by the time constant of the patient's lungs. As illustrated in Fig. 5.13, a high airway resistance leads to a large time constant and necessitates a prolonged period to allow expiration of the tidal volume whereas, in the case of a low compliance, the time constant is reduced and a short period of expiration suffices with a more rapid respiratory rate.

In the case of a washout curve, the time constant can be shown mathematically to be equal to the volume undergoing washout divided by the flow of the perfusing fluid:

$$\tau = \frac{\text{Volume undergoing washout}}{\text{Flow of perfusing fluid}}$$

The time constant may be obtained from analysis of a washout curve and if the volume undergoing washout is also known, the flow of the perfusing fluid may be calculated. Conversely, the volume undergoing washout can be calculated if the time constant and flow of the perfusing fluid are known. Many methods of measuring blood flow in organs are based on this principle. Radioactive isotopes are often used for such measurements, a radioactive isotope being injected into the organ and the rate at which it is washed out by the blood measured by a scintillation counter (Chapter 24). From this, the time constant is found. As this time constant is proportional to the volume divided by the flow, if volume is known, flow can be calculated.

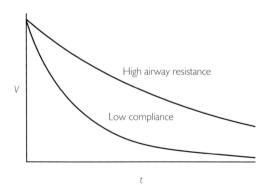

Figure 5.13 Plot of expired gas volume as a function of time in a patient with a high airway resistance and in a patient with a low compliance

It has previously been noted that the characteristic of an exponential process is the proportionality between a quantity and its rate of change, i.e.

$$\dot{Q} \propto Q$$

An expression of proportionality like this can also be written as

$$\dot{Q} = kQ$$

where k is known as the constant of proportionality. It can be shown mathematically that the constant of proportionality is the reciprocal of the time constant, i.e.

$$k = \frac{1}{\tau}$$

The reciprocal, k, of the time constant is known as the rate constant, and is sometimes used as an alternative.

The Exponential Formula

Now that the exponential type of function has been described, the exponential formula may be considered. The word exponential arises from the exponent or index, which is in superscript below:

fixed exponent   variable exponent
$y = x^2$ $y = k^x$

On the left is an equation or function with a fixed exponent (2 in the example), and on the right is a function with a variable exponent x. The latter is an exponential function.

In medicine, the type of exponential function encountered is normally one in which the rate of change of the quantity is proportional to the quantity at that time, as described earlier. This is called a natural exponential function, and the constant k in the above equation has a special value of 2.718. In mathematics this quantity 2.718 is given the symbol e. The exponential formula which describes the emptying of a lung is as follows:

$$V_t = V_0 \, e^{-t/CR}$$

where V_t is the volume at t seconds, V_0 is the volume at zero seconds, e is 2.718, C is the compliance and R is the resistance.

The volumes V are the volumes of air in the lungs in excess of the functional residual capacity. In this case, e is raised to the power of $-t/CR$ and the fact that the exponent has a negative value indicates that, as time increases, the value of V_t steadily decreases. Such a negative exponent is characteristic of a negative exponential function.

The Positive Exponential Process

So far, only negative exponential processes have been considered, but positive exponential processes also exist, as shown in Fig. 5.14.

In this case, the process is increasing at a faster and faster rate, but at any time the rate of change is proportional to the quantity at that time. An example of a positive exponential curve is bacterial growth in the presence of unlimited nutrient and in some cases the multiplication of cancer cells may initially follow a similar pattern.

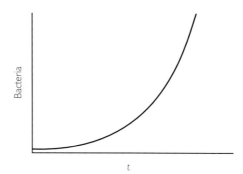

Figure 5.14 Positive exponential process

The Build-Up Exponential Process

These positive exponential curves must not be confused with another type of exponential, the build-up exponential (Fig. 5.15), which is more relevant to anaesthesia than the positive form.

In this case, the curve appears like an inverted negative exponential. The exponential component of the process is the difference between the value achieved and the eventual theoretical final value. This difference is represented by shading in Fig. 5.15.

Figure 5.16 shows a bath as an illustration of a build-up exponential process. The bath on the right is being filled through its plug hole from a constant head of water in a large reservoir on the left. In this case, the rate of filling of the bath at any time depends on the difference, Δh, between the height of the water in the bath and the eventual value it will achieve. This height, Δh, is proportional to the pressure driving the water through the connecting tube.

As an example of a build-up exponential in anaesthesia, consider the inflation of the lungs with a constant-pressure ventilator (Fig. 5.17). In the ventilator on the left, the weight acting over the area of the bellows gives rise to the constant pressure. In this case, the inflation of the lungs is rapid initially but slows as the lungs reach full inflation. From the analogy with the washout curves discussed earlier, these build-up exponentials are sometimes known as 'washin' curves and this concept is particularly helpful to the understanding of the induction of anaesthesia. Such anaesthetic uptake curves are closely analogous to the elimination curves, except that they are inverted.

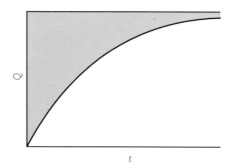

Figure 5.15 Build-up exponential process

Figure 5.16 A bath as an analogy for the build-up exponential process

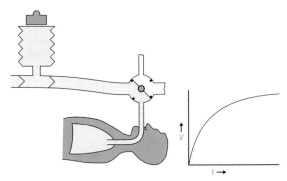

Figure 5.17 Inflation of the lungs by a constant-pressure ventilator

The uptake of an anaesthetic, however, is not strictly speaking a simple single exponential process, but one consisting of many exponentials. Ventilation is one exponential process because it carries the inspired anaesthetic to the lungs; a further exponential process involves the circulation, where the anaesthetic is carried from the lungs to the tissues.

Figure 5.18 illustrates this in terms of the filling of reservoirs of liquid. However, this is a simplified illustration as, in fact, there is not just one tissue, represented by the reservoir on the right, but many with different rates of exponential uptake of the anaesthetic. Elimination of a volatile anaesthetic is in the reverse direction and, again, it comprises several exponential processes.

A complex process, such as the uptake or excretion of anaesthetic, may be separated mathematically into its component parts. If a multiple exponential process is plotted on semilogarithmic graph paper, a curve is obtained on the graph

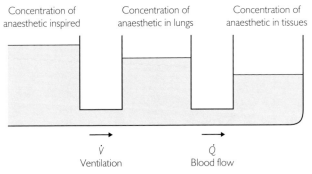

Figure 5.18 A simplified bath analogy for the uptake of an inspired anaesthetic agent into the lungs and tissues

instead of the straight line of a simple exponential. This curve can then be analysed and broken down, as shown in Fig. 5.19.

In this simple example, the curve is found to be composed of three exponential processes (A, B and C), each giving one straight line. Normally, a computer is used to analyse such curves. Other aspects of the uptake and excretion of anaesthetics are considered in Chapter 6.

Another example of a multiple exponential process is the absorption of an orally administered drug from the gut into the plasma, followed by the excretion of the drug from the bloodstream. In a simple model of this process, the drug can be considered as passing out through two compartments: the gut and the plasma. The rate at which the drug leaves the gut is proportional to the quantity of drug in the gut; similarly, the rate at which the drug leaves the bloodstream is proportional to the quantity of drug in the plasma. Consequently, the concentration of drug in the gut decreases exponentially with time. However, the situation in the blood is more complex, as the drug is both entering the bloodstream through absorption from the gut and leaving the bloodstream by metabolism or excretion. The concentration in the plasma is therefore a curve composed of two exponentials: the double exponential curve shown in Fig. 5.20.

If oral doses of a drug are administered sequentially, the concentrations in the gut and in the bloodstream increase and decrease as shown in Fig. 5.21. The dose

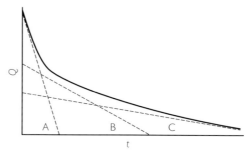

Figure 5.19 A complex process consisting of three exponentials – A, B and C in the graph – can be analysed into its components

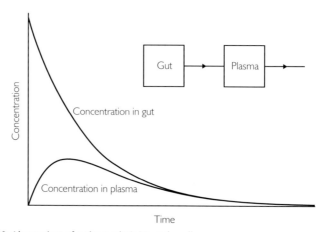

Figure 5.20 Absorption of a drug administered orally

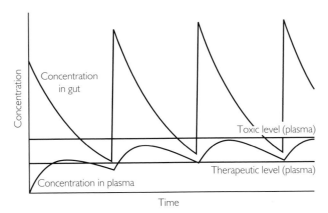

Figure 5.21 Changes in plasma concentration of a drug associated with repeated oral doses

and the frequency at which the drug is taken must be chosen to avoid the plasma concentration decreasing below the therapeutic level or increasing above the toxic level. A less-variable blood level can be achieved by infusing the drug at a steady rate using an infusion or syringe pump.

Solubility

6

The Concept of Solubility

As explained in Chapter 4, when a liquid is placed in a closed container an equilibrium is eventually established at the surface between the vapour of the liquid and the liquid itself. In this equilibrium state, the partial pressure exerted by the vapour is known as the saturated vapour pressure. In practice, there is usually at least one gas present above the surface of the liquid in addition to the vapour.

In Fig. 6.1, molecules of a liquid and its vapour are shown as open circles, and molecules of a gas are shown as black dots. An occasional molecule of gas above the surface passes into solution in the liquid as indicated at Y. In addition, molecules of dissolved gas in the liquid occasionally leave, as indicated at X. Eventually an equilibrium occurs when dissolved gas molecules leave the liquid at the same rate at which others dissolve. In this condition, the liquid and the dissolved gas are said to form a saturated solution. As an example, the liquid could be water and the gas molecules could be nitrogen.

On the left of Fig. 6.2, the gas is at a normal atmospheric pressure of 100 kPa (1 bar) and in equilibrium with the liquid below. On the right, the pressure is doubled to a hyperbaric level of 200 kPa (2 bar); hence there are twice as many molecules of gas above the water, resulting in twice as many in solution, as illustrated. The amount of nitrogen dissolved in water, for example, is proportional to the pressure of nitrogen above the water. Note, however, that the temperature must be kept constant for this to apply. This principle is known as Henry's law:

Gas + vapour

Gas in solution + liquid

Figure 6.1 Molecular equilibrium at the surface of a liquid

Figure 6.2 Effect of pressure on the amount of gas dissolved in a liquid

Henry's law states that at a particular temperature the amount of a given gas dissolved in a given liquid is directly proportional to the partial pressure of the gas in equilibrium with the liquid.

The effect of high pressure on the solubility of nitrogen is particularly relevant to deep-sea divers, as nitrogen and other gases, if breathed under pressure, pass into solution in the tissues. If a return to atmospheric pressure is made too rapidly, the nitrogen comes out of solution as small bubbles in the joints and elsewhere, giving rise to the condition known as decompression sickness or 'the bends'. Similar problems apply to workers in hyperbaric chambers, where again a decompression that is too rapid can lead to 'the bends'.

Henry's law applies only if the temperature is constant. Consider now what happens if the temperature is altered. Figure 6.3 shows two measuring cylinders, each containing 1 litre of water and exposed in an atmosphere of nitrogen. The left cylinder is at a room temperature of 20°C, the right one at body temperature, 37°C. The pressure of the nitrogen in both cases is 100 kPa, but the volume of nitrogen that is dissolved in the litre of water in the cylinder at room temperature is 0.016 litre, whereas at body temperature it is only 0.014 litre. It is a general property that as a liquid is warmed, less gas dissolves in it. In a kettle about to boil, the simmering which occurs is due to the release of bubbles of air which come out of solution as the water is heated. Similarly, in the operating theatre, bubbles of air

Figure 6.3 Effect of temperature on the amount of gas dissolved in a liquid

Figure 6.4 Effect of the gas concerned on solubility

may form in saline in an infusion line which has passed through a blood-warming coil.

Consider now what happens if a gas other than nitrogen is used. The measuring cylinder on the left of Fig. 6.4 contains 1 litre of water in an atmosphere of nitrogen and on the right is a similar cylinder in an atmosphere of nitrous oxide. At equilibrium there is considerably more nitrous oxide dissolved in the litre of water than in the case of nitrogen: 0.39 litre of nitrous oxide compared with 0.014 litre of nitrogen. So different gases are found to have different solubilities.

Finally, the liquid too must be specified when considering solubility. As shown in Fig. 6.5, 0.39 litre of nitrous oxide dissolves in 1 litre of water at body temperature, whereas 1 litre of blood dissolves 0.47 litre of nitrous oxide under the same conditions. To summarize, the solubility of a gas depends on the partial pressure, the temperature, the gas and the liquid concerned.

Solubility Coefficients

The solubility of solids is described in terms of a given number of moles or millimoles of the solute which dissolve in 1 litre of the solvent, but for gases it is, in practice, much easier to express a quantity in terms of its volume, as in the previous examples. The volume of a gas, however, only has an accurate meaning if the pressure and temperature are specified, and for scientific work the volume of a gas is normally corrected to STP. Physicists therefore use a solubility coefficient, known as the Bunsen solubility coefficient, which uses such a correction:

The Bunsen solubility coefficient is the volume of gas, corrected to STP, which dissolves in 1 unit volume of the liquid at the temperature concerned, where the partial pressure of the gas above the liquid is 1 standard atmosphere pressure.

The Bunsen coefficient is the solubility coefficient usually quoted in scientific tables and textbooks but in anaesthetic practice another solubility coefficient is preferred. This is known as the Ostwald solubility coefficient:

The Ostwald solubility coefficient is the volume of gas which dissolves in 1 unit volume of the liquid at the temperature concerned.

The volume of gas is not corrected to standard temperature and pressure in this case but, instead, is measured at a known temperature and pressure. The practical advantage of the Ostwald solubility coefficient is that it is independent of pressure.

Figure 6.5 Effect of the liquid concerned on the solubility of a gas

Figure 6.6 illustrates this independence of pressure. On the left, there is 100 kPa pressure (1 bar) of nitrogen above the surface of 1 litre of water. A volume of 0.016 litre of nitrogen at that pressure dissolves in the water. On the right, there is a pressure of 200 kPa (2 bar) of nitrogen above the water. Consider what happens. According to Henry's law, the quantity of the gas dissolving is proportional to the pressure, so there is twice as much nitrogen dissolved in the water on the right: i.e. 0.032 litre if measured at a pressure of 100 kPa. But when this volume is measured at the ambient pressure of 2 bar, it is half this value: i.e. 0.016 litre (Boyle's law). Consequently, the volume of nitrogen dissolved measured at the ambient pressure remains constant even though the partial pressure of the nitrogen is doubled and the number of nitrogen molecules in solution is also doubled. The Ostwald solubility coefficient does not therefore need to be defined in terms of pressure because pressure does not modify the volume which dissolves, provided that the volume is measured at the ambient pressure.

Figure 6.6 The illustration shows that the Ostwald solubility coefficient is independent of pressure

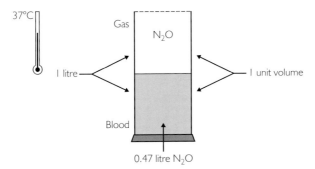

Figure 6.7 Partition coefficient

The Partition Coefficient

The partition coefficient is similar to the Ostwald solubility coefficient. To understand the term partition coefficient, consider the example of nitrous oxide and blood shown in Fig. 6.7. There is a unit volume of 1 litre of nitrous oxide above the same unit volume of 1 litre of blood which contains dissolved nitrous oxide in equilibrium at 37°C. The volume of nitrous oxide dissolved in these circumstances is 0.47 litre and the ratio of 0.47 to 1 is the blood–gas partition coefficient for nitrous oxide.

The partition coefficient is defined as the ratio of the amount of substance present in one phase compared with another, the two phases being of equal volume and in equilibrium.

As with the Ostwald solubility coefficient, the temperature should be specified and, in addition, the phases concerned must be stated. In Fig 6.7 the temperature is 37°C, the phases are blood and gas, and the nitrous oxide blood–gas partition coefficient is 0.47, the same as the Ostwald solubility coefficient. Notice, however, the relative order of the phases of the partition coefficient must be clearly identified. For instance, if the nitrous oxide gas–blood coefficient were specified instead of the blood–gas coefficient, the value would be 2.1 instead of 0.47, as 2.1 is the reciprocal of 0.47.

Another difference between the partition coefficient and the Ostwald solubility coefficient is that the former can be applied to two liquids.

Figure 6.8 shows an illustration with two liquids, blood and oil. At equilibrium, the ratio of the amount of nitrous oxide present in unit volume of blood to that in unit volume of oil is the blood–oil partition coefficient. In this case, 1.4 litres of nitrous oxide dissolves in 1 litre of oil, compared with 0.47 litre in 1 litre of blood. Thus, the blood–oil partition coefficient for nitrous oxide is 0.47/1.4, or 0.33. In the case of partition coefficients, the nitrous oxide or other dissolved gas must be in equilibrium in the two phases: i.e. the tension must be the same in the two phases.

The word tension is often used in place of partial pressure for gases in solution and Fig. 6.9 shows the pressure or partial pressure of nitrous oxide in the gaseous phase above blood as 50 kPa. When in equilibrium, the tension of nitrous oxide in the blood is also 50 kPa. The tension of a gas in solution is the partial pressure of the gas which would be in equilibrium with it. The word tension is also used in physics in another sense when referring to forces (Chapter 1).

Figure 6.8 Application of the partition coefficient to two liquids

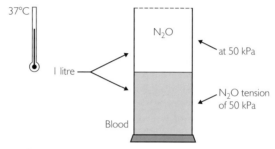

Figure 6.9 Tension of a gas

Solubility and Uptake of Anaesthetics

Some clinical applications of solubility may now be considered.

Figure 6.10 shows three measuring cylinders, all containing 1 litre of blood at a temperature of 37°C and exposed to an atmosphere of nitrous oxide, halothane and ether, respectively. There are many more molecules of ether present in the blood because it has the highest Ostwald solubility coefficient (12), which is higher than halothane (2.3) or nitrous oxide (0.47).

How does the increased solubility of the ether affect the rate at which it can be transported away from the lungs in the blood? Because it is much more soluble, ether is carried away from the lungs more rapidly than halothane or nitrous

Figure 6.10 Solubility of anaesthetic agents in blood

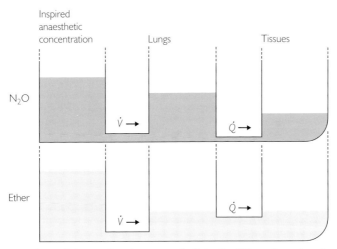

Figure 6.11 Analogy of the uptake of an anaesthetic to the filling of a series of reservoirs

oxide and hence the concentration of ether in the alveolar air builds up more slowly than that of a less-soluble anaesthetic.

As explained in Chapter 5, the uptake of an anaesthetic can be represented diagrammatically by a set of reservoirs, and Fig. 6.11 shows such a system to illustrate the effect of solubility. The reservoir on the left represents the inspired anaesthetic concentration. The transport of the anaesthetic to the lungs by the ventilation is represented by the pipe joining it to the second reservoir and the ventilation is indicated by $\dot{V}$. The second or central reservoir represents the lungs, i.e. the concentration of anaesthetic in the alveolar air. The removal of the anaesthetic by the pulmonary blood flow from this reservoir is denoted by the next pipe and the rate of transport by the cardiac output is shown as $\dot{Q}$. The right reservoir represents the tissues.

The upper part of Fig. 6.11 illustrates the uptake of nitrous oxide. The central reservoir represents the alveolar concentration of the anaesthetic, and its narrow outlet pipe indicates that the anaesthetic can be carried away only relatively slowly by the cardiac output because the solubility coefficient of nitrous oxide is only 0.47.

The lower part of Fig. 6.11 shows what happens when ether is used. The high solubility of ether in the blood means that it can be carried away from the lungs very rapidly. This is indicated by the very wide pipe and the high value of $\dot{Q}$ and, in consequence, the alveolar concentration of ether is only slightly above the tissue concentration.

Figure 6.12 illustrates the build-up exponential curves produced if alveolar concentrations of anaesthetics are expressed as percentages of their final values and plotted against time. It is seen that soluble anaesthetics such as ether are very slow to approach their final value, whereas equilibrium is approached in 10–15 min with nitrous oxide. Because the concentrations of anaesthetics in the blood and brain are close to the alveolar concentrations, there is a rapid onset of anaesthesia in the case of nitrous oxide and a relatively slower induction of anaesthesia with ether.

In these illustrations, nitrous oxide has been represented as an agent of low solubility, but solubility is relative and nitrous oxide is much more soluble than

Figure 6.12 Alveolar concentrations of anaesthetics versus time during anaesthetic uptake

nitrogen. Consider the instance in which a simple pattern of a Benedict Roth spirometer is used to measure the volume of a gas mixture containing nitrous oxide, oxygen and nitrogen.

As shown in Fig. 6.13, more nitrous oxide passes into solution than oxygen or nitrogen and this could lead to a slight error, although with the small volume of water in the water seal of such spirometers, this error is minimal. A greater loss of nitrous oxide into solution would have an effect on the concentrations of the other gases, oxygen and nitrogen, in the bell of the spirometer, resulting in a rise in the concentrations of oxygen and nitrogen. A similar effect occurs in the alveoli during induction of anaesthesia. During the course of an inspiration of a gas mixture containing nitrous oxide, the nitrous oxide is absorbed into the bloodstream faster than the oxygen or nitrogen, so at peak inspiration, when the pressure in the alveoli has equalized with the ambient pressure, there is a net surplus of oxygen and nitrogen molecules. This phenomenon is called the second-gas effect and is important when considering the uptake of anaesthetic agents.

A similar phenomenon occurs during the excretion of nitrous oxide at the end of anaesthesia when nitrous oxide leaving the blood and entering the alveoli dilutes the gases already present. The fall of oxygen concentration thus produced is known as diffusion hypoxia.

Figure 6.13 Potential error in volume measurement due to gas solubility in a water seal

Figure 6.14 Solubilities of anaesthetic agents in oil

Figure 6.15 Minimum alveolar concentration (MAC) and oil solubility coefficients of anaesthetic agents.

Oil Solubility and Anaesthetic Potency

Fat is an important constituent of many body tissues, being present in cell membranes and neurones in particular. Fat and oil are very similar and, because it is easier to measure solubilities in oil, it is oil that is normally used for measurements.

Figure 6.14 illustrates the relative solubilities of nitrous oxide, ether and halothane in oil: the greater the solubility, the greater the number of dots representing the molecules of anaesthetic agent in the oil. The solubilities in oil are in a different order from those in blood (Fig. 6.10). Although nitrous oxide is still the least soluble, the agent with the greatest solubility is now halothane as shown on the right, ether being midway between nitrous oxide and halothane.

Agents that have the highest oil solubility are found to have the greatest potency as anaesthetics and this was the basis of the Meyer–Overton theory of anaesthesia, illustrated in a modified form in Fig. 6.15.

The vertical axis of the graph is the MAC (minimum alveolar concentration) for the anaesthetic, the MAC value being the point at which 50% of patients cease to move in response to a stimulus. On the horizontal axis are the oil solubility coefficients of the anaesthetics and in order to cover the range of anaesthetics, a logarithmic scale has been used. When plotted in this way the anaesthetics are found to lie on a straight line and from the slope of the line it is seen that an anaesthetic with a high solubility in oil has a low MAC value. In other words, an anaesthetic with a high oil solubility is effective at a low alveolar concentration and has a high potency.

An alternative way of expressing this principle is to say that the MAC value for any anaesthetic is related to the number of molecules of anaesthetic dissolved in oil, and this applies to all volatile anaesthetics. The MAC value of over 100% for nitrous oxide shown in Fig. 6.15 is, of course, a theoretical one based on the partial pressure of nitrous oxide when used for anaesthesia in a pressure chamber.

To explain the interrelation of the potency of anaesthetics and their solubility in oil, the high solubility of potent anaesthetics is thought to be associated with a mild attraction of the anaesthetic molecules to those of fatty acid chains. Anaesthetics may act at some point in the brain by interfering with the molecular configuration of the long fatty acid or similar molecular chains at a critical point within the neurones or their synapses. The attachment of the anaesthetic molecules to the chain molecules is relatively loose and readily reversible with van der Waals type bonds.

Anaesthetic molecules are also attracted to the long carbon chain molecules present in rubber and plastics. The solubility of anaesthetic agents in rubber and in some plastics results in changes in the physical properties of these materials and this has practical importance in anaesthesia. Substantial quantities of anaesthetics may be absorbed into the tubing used in breathing systems, and the more soluble the anaesthetic in the tubing, the greater the volume which is absorbed in this way. Potent anaesthetic agents such as isoflurane, for example, can be absorbed in considerable quantities and trace amounts of these anaesthetics may later be released and administered to patients even if no anaesthetic vaporizer is turned on.

Although the concentrations of anaesthetic agents released in this way are generally small, the quantity may be sufficient to trigger the onset of malignant hyperpyrexia. Any patient who is at risk from this syndrome should therefore receive anaesthesia only from equipment from which all possible sources of absorbed anaesthetic vapour have been removed.

Diffusion and Osmosis

7

Diffusion is the process by which the molecules of a substance transfer through a layer or area such as the surface of a solution. In the lungs, gases diffuse across a gas–liquid barrier in this way, but diffusion may also occur at other sites, shown diagrammatically in Fig. 7.1.

The diffusion of gases in the body is illustrated by compartments in the form of layers in a bottle. At the top, gas in the alveoli of the lungs is represented and below it the alveolar–capillary membrane where the gas diffuses into the liquid phase, i.e. the blood. There are then further membranes at which diffusion occurs – between the blood and the extracellular fluid and between the extracellular fluid and the cell – allowing the gas to pass from one compartment of the body to the next.

Diffusion can still take place without a membrane or a gas–liquid barrier. For example, if gas escapes from a broken gas pipe, the gas spreads by diffusion even after the gas tap has been turned off.

Factors Affecting the Rate of Diffusion

Figure 7.2 provides an example in which two different concentrations of a substance or gas diffuse into a region of lower concentration. This could represent the gas from the broken pipe in the example above, or an anaesthetic agent diffusing across a membrane, or a gas diffusing into a liquid. On the right, the concentration is double that on the left and it is found that the rate of diffusion through the surface or membrane is doubled. If there is a gas concentration below the membrane, an allowance for this must be made and the rate of diffusion would depend on the concentration gradient across the membrane.

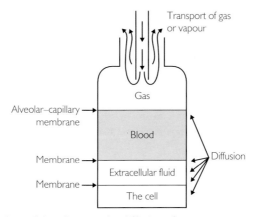

Figure 7.1 Simple model to illustrate the diffusion of a gas or vapour in the body

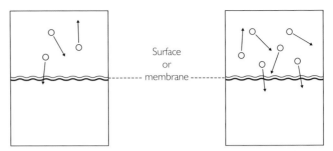

Figure 7.2 Effect of concentration on the rate of diffusion

The law defining this relationship is Fick's law of diffusion:

Fick's law states that the rate of diffusion of a substance across unit area (such as a surface or membrane) is proportional to the concentration gradient.

Fick's law applies only in a single homogeneous phase and a slight modification is needed if gases are transferring from one phase into another, as in the case of gases passing into solution. The modified form of the law is that the rate of diffusion of a gas across a membrane (or surface area) is proportional to the tension gradient.

The tension of a gas in solution describes the partial pressure of the gas which would be in equilibrium with it, as explained in Chapter 6. For convenience the word tension is often used instead of partial pressure for the gas in the gaseous phase. This modified form of Fick's law is more relevant in anaesthesia than the original form because it applies universally. For example, it is relevant to clinical situations in which a membrane or interface exists between gases, or between liquids, or between gas and liquid.

These laws apply only to a given gas and a given membrane because different gases have different rates of diffusion, and membranes also vary in their diffusing capacity.

Fick's law of diffusion may now be considered in the context of the transport to the cell of a gas or vapour. At the top of Fig. 7.1 inspired gas is illustrated being transported by ventilation and at this point the rate at which the gas is transported would be the flow multiplied by the concentration. Once the gas reaches the alveolar–capillary membrane, diffusion takes place, and here the tension gradient is important. In the circulation, again there is mass transport, the rate being flow times concentration, but from the blood to the cell there are two membranes with the extracellular fluid compartment between them. Diffusion takes place at these points and so the rate is affected by the tissue tension gradients. In addition to diffusion at these points, however, the carriage of the gases may also be helped by fluid movements in the extracellular fluid caused by osmosis (discussed later).

The same patterns of diffusion and mass transport apply in reverse for a substance such as carbon dioxide which is produced at the cell and excreted by the ventilation.

Consider now diffusion across the alveolar–capillary membrane (Fig. 7.3). Here the gas passes into the liquid phase and, once in solution, diffusion of the gas depends on the tension or concentration gradients in the liquid itself. The greater the solubility of the gas in the liquid, the greater will be the concentration gradient between the surface layer of the liquid and its deeper layers; hence a more soluble gas diffuses into the deeper layers of the liquid more rapidly. This

Figure 7.3 Diffusion across the alveolar–capillary membrane

maintains a tension gradient between the gas and the surface layer of the liquid and increases the rate of diffusion of the gas into the liquid. The diffusion of a gas across a membrane into or out of a liquid is thus proportional to its solubility in the liquid.

Figure 7.4 illustrates this diffusion process for carbon dioxide and oxygen. Because carbon dioxide is more soluble in tissue fluid than oxygen, it diffuses more rapidly. Below the diagrams, graphs illustrate the rate of diffusion across the alveolar–capillary membrane for carbon dioxide and oxygen. The blood normally takes 0.75 s to pass through the capillary, but carbon dioxide equilibrates virtually instantaneously in less than 0.1 s. Oxygen equilibrium is normally complete by the time the blood has passed half the way down the capillary. The longer time taken for the oxygen is due to two factors: slower diffusion compared with carbon dioxide and the removal of the oxygen molecules from the plasma as they combine with haemoglobin in the red cells. If diffusing capacity is limited, hypoxia is thus more likely to occur than hypercapnia. Nevertheless, there is still a reserve of time for oxygen to reach equilibrium before the blood leaves the capillary and mild limitation of diffusion does not normally produce symptoms.

The diffusion of volatile anaesthetic agents resembles carbon dioxide – equilibrium being complete within a small fraction of a second – and so diffusion is ignored in Chapter 6 when considering the uptake of anaesthetics.

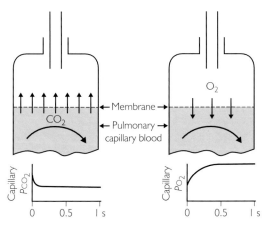

Figure 7.4 Diffusion of carbon dioxide and oxygen

Pulmonary Diffusing Capacity and Carbon Monoxide Transfer Test

Diffusion across the alveolar–capillary membrane is altered by certain diseases and can be measured by a method using carbon monoxide. This measurement, known as the pulmonary diffusing capacity or transfer test, is the rate of carbon monoxide uptake, standardized according to the tension gradient. Because carbon monoxide is very toxic, it can be used only in trace amounts, but a patient can safely inhale a carbon monoxide concentration of 0.1% into the alveoli for a short period. As haemoglobin has a high affinity for carbon monoxide, the carbon monoxide molecules combine rapidly with the cells in the bloodstream and are carried away. Consequently, it would take a very long time for the plasma in the pulmonary capillaries to equilibrate with the alveolar gas and produce a significant carbon monoxide tension. The carbon monoxide tension in the pulmonary capillaries during this test can therefore be regarded as zero. The rate at which the carbon monoxide leaves the alveoli is therefore dependent on the rate of diffusion through the membrane and not on the pulmonary blood flow. In this way the rate of uptake of trace concentrations of carbon monoxide is used to measure diffusing capacity.

As lungs have a large reserve of diffusing capacity, small reductions are of little importance in patients. For example, a pneumonectomy halves the available membrane area and so approximately halves the diffusing capacity, but even a pneumonectomy does not normally give rise to any serious problems from this reduction of diffusing capacity. Certain diseases, however, such as sarcoidosis, asbestosis and sometimes systemic lupus erythematosus, affect the alveolar–capillary membrane itself and can give rise to a severe reduction of diffusing capacity. Thus, the measurement of the diffusing capacity may be of value in the diagnosis of these diseases.

As illustrated in Fig. 7.1, there are further membrane barriers between the blood in the capillaries and the extracellular fluid, and between the extracellular fluid and the cells. Diffusing capacity is altered if oedema is present, because oedema fluid impairs the diffusion of gases or other agents to the cells by increasing the distance from the capillary to the cell surface.

Practical Aspects of Diffusion

Consider now some practical points regarding diffusion and anaesthetic apparatus. Anaesthetic systems deliver isoflurane vapour through corrugated rubber tubing and, as isoflurane is soluble in rubber, it diffuses readily into and through the rubber of the tube. The rubber tube thus provides a possible source from which isoflurane may diffuse into the theatre atmosphere, in addition to the more direct route from release of isoflurane vapour through the expiratory valve. As mentioned in Chapter 6, isoflurane may remain stored in the rubber due to its high solubility, and trace levels may be released later.

As another example of the effect of tension gradients on diffusion, consider a patient with decompression sickness in whom bubbles of nitrogen form in the tissues.

On the left of Fig. 7.5 is a bubble of nitrogen in the tissues within a capillary loop. If the patient then receives anaesthesia with 50% nitrous oxide, a tension gradient develops as shown and the arterial tension of nitrous oxide could be 50 kPa compared with zero tension within the bubble. Nitrous oxide diffuses into

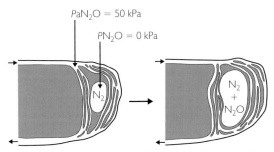

$PaN_2O = 50$ kPa

$PN_2O = 0$ kPa

Figure 7.5 Effect of nitrous oxide on the size of a bubble of nitrogen in the tissues

the bubble, thus enlarging it – as shown on the right of Fig. 7.5 – and aggravates the condition. The problem is not limited to patients with decompression sickness but applies equally to those with bubbles of air at other sites such as a pneumothorax. Even air in the middle ear expands and this may give rise to problems in grafts in that region. In Fig. 7.5 there is a reverse gradient for nitrogen, but the nitrogen is not removed from the bubble at the same rate that nitrous oxide diffuses into it because the lower solubility of nitrogen restricts the rate of its diffusion and the rate at which the capillary bloodstream removes it. Another example of nitrous oxide diffusion arises routinely during the course of anaesthesia, when the gas diffuses into the cuff of an endotracheal tube, so increasing the pressure on the tracheal mucosa.

Effect of Molecular Size

Consider now the effect of varying the size of the molecules of the substance which is diffusing.

In Fig. 7.6 there is a broken ether bottle on the floor of a room in which ventilation is negligible; the ether vapour has formed a smooth layer over the floor, ether being more dense than air. On the right, a gas pipe has broken and has released hydrogen into the upper part of the room. Because small molecules move faster than large molecules at the same temperature, the hydrogen diffuses more rapidly than the ether and the ether vapour tends to remain longer as a layer.

The relationship of the molecular size to the rate of diffusion is defined by Graham's law of diffusion:

Graham's law states that the rate of diffusion of a gas is inversely proportional to the square root of its molecular weight.

Ether vapour

Hydrogen gas

Broken gas pipe

Tap

Broken ether bottle

Figure 7.6 Effect of molecular size on diffusion rate

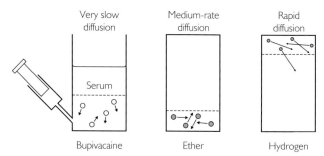

Figure 7.7 Diffusion in a liquid, e.g. serum, is slower than in a vapour or gas

When dealing with membranes, the law applies only in certain cases and it does not apply accurately when more complex biological membranes are involved. Although Graham's law applies to gases, the concept that the rate of diffusion is related to molecular size may also be applied to liquids.

On the left of Fig. 7.7 bupivacaine is shown, injected underneath a layer of serum so that it forms a smooth layer. The molecular movement in liquids is much slower and more limited than in the case of gases, and this is illustrated in the diagram by the shorter arrows. There is a very slow rate of diffusion in liquids such as serum compared with the rate of diffusion in vapours or gases. When injecting local anaesthetics into the tissues it is important to inject the anaesthetic close to the nerves concerned, because diffusion allows only limited penetration of the local anaesthetic into the tissues. In the case of cerebrospinal fluid there are also convection currents and gravitational effects depending on the density of the local anaesthetic. All these effects help the local anaesthetic to reach the appropriate nerve roots.

The main points regarding diffusion may be summarized as follows. Diffusion is proportional to the tension gradient and, because solubility has a pronounced effect on tension gradients, this in turn affects the rate of diffusion. Diffusion also depends on the membrane concerned, its area, thickness and its constituents. Finally, diffusion is affected by the molecular size, the larger-sized molecules diffusing less rapidly than smaller ones and liquids diffusing less rapidly than gases.

Osmosis

Consider now a membrane that does not allow the passage of all molecules: i.e. a semipermeable membrane, separating a solution from a solvent, as shown in Fig. 7.8.

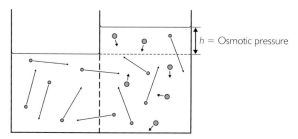

Figure 7.8 Principle of osmosis

The small molecules of solvent can readily pass through the membrane, but in the compartment on the right there are some large solute molecules which cannot pass through. In this compartment the concentration of small solvent molecules is reduced by the presence of the solute. If Fick's law of diffusion is applied, what would happen to the small molecules? They diffuse from the area of higher concentration on the left across to the right side, giving a transfer of liquid. If the transfer is allowed to continue long enough, equilibrium is achieved and then 'h', the excess height of the compartment on the right, represents the osmotic pressure. It is the pressure which exactly counterbalances the effect of the dissolved molecules. An alternative way of achieving equilibrium is to have a closed compartment, as shown in Fig. 7.9.

If the compartment on the right has a 22.4-litre capacity, and if it contains 1 mol of particles of solute at a temperature of 0°C, then the osmotic pressure built up in this compartment is 101.325 kPa or 1 standard atmosphere. This is shown in the diagram by the gauge pressure, this being additional to the ambient pressure also present. Note that this is similar to the concept that 1 mol of a perfect gas in a volume of 22.4 litres exerts a pressure of 1 atmosphere (Chapter 4). Provided that 1 mol of solute is present in the compartment and that the membrane is not permeable to the solute molecules, the size of these molecules is immaterial.

In clinical practice there are many different types of molecules present in plasma, urine or other body fluids. In order to distinguish between the molarity of individual specific components and the sum total of molarities which give rise to the osmotic pressure, the term 'osmolarity' is used. As an example consider the components of Ringer's lactate solution.

Sodium 131 mmol litre^{-1}
Potassium 5 mmol litre^{-1}
Calcium 2 mmol litre^{-1}
Lactate* 29 mmol litre^{-1}
Chloride 111 mmol litre^{-1}
Total osmolarity 278 mosmol litre^{-1}

*Assuming the lactate is all in ionized form

Each component is present in various concentrations of mmol litre^{-1}, but it is the sum total of the molarities which gives rise to the osmotic pressure. In other words, the osmolarity of the solution is the sum of the molarities of the solutes. In Ringer's lactate solution, the total osmolarity is 278 mosmol litre^{-1}.

0°C

101.325 kPa
(1 atmosphere)

1 mole of particles of solute in 22.4 litre

Figure 7.9 An osmotic pressure of 101.325 kPa is produced when 1 mol solute is dissolved in 22.4 litres of solution at 0°C

Figure 7.10 Pressure balance in a capillary loop

Most body fluids such as plasma have an osmolarity of about 300 mosmol litre^{-1}. Over 99% of the osmolarity of plasma is due to electrolytes such as sodium, chloride and bicarbonate; the contribution of the plasma proteins is very small at around 1 mosmol litre^{-1}. Most fluids administered to the patient are adjusted to have an osmolarity of around 300 mosmol litre^{-1}. This means that they are isotonic with body fluids. If a patient is transfused with fluids of low osmolarity, i.e. hypotonic fluids, then the change in the osmotic pressure gradient across the cell membranes causes fluid to diffuse into the cells, giving a rise of hydrostatic pressure in them.

Use is made of this fact in the red cell fragility test for the detection of haemolytic anaemias. Red cells are added to various concentrations of saline at 20°C. The lower the osmolarity of the solution, the greater the hydrostatic pressure which builds up in the red cells as fluid passes into them. Thus, at osmolarities below 200 mosmol litre^{-1}, the red cells burst and release haemoglobin into the solution. In many haemolytic anaemias the red cells are abnormal and more fragile and so burst at higher osmolarities than normal.

The main difference between plasma and interstitial fluid is the relative proportions of protein, the proportion being negligible in the latter. As the membrane of blood capillaries is permeable to water and electrolytes but not to large protein molecules, the osmotic pressure between the blood and extracellular fluid depends on the protein molecules. To distinguish this pressure from total osmotic pressure it is sometimes called the oncotic pressure. Although albumin and globulin in the plasma have a very small osmolarity of around 1 mosmol litre^{-1}, they give rise to an oncotic pressure in the capillaries of about 3.5 kPa (26 mmHg), the pressure being principally due to the albumin because of its higher molar concentration.

Figure 7.10 illustrates a capillary loop with an arterial pressure of 7 kPa (53 mmHg) and a venous pressure near to zero. The balance of pressures is closely related to the oncotic pressure from the plasma proteins. Thus, at the arterial end of the capillary, the hydrostatic pressure exceeds the oncotic pressure by 3.5 kPa and this results in the passage of fluid out of the capillary. At the venous end the pressure ratios are reversed and tissue fluid therefore passes into the capillary. These pressure gradients produce a continual fluid flow through the tissues to help carry oxygen and carbon dioxide and other agents to and from the cells. This is an important mechanism because diffusion alone does not enable solutes to move rapidly through a liquid. The example is simplified as the small hydrostatic and oncotic pressures in the tissue fluid have been disregarded.

A fall of plasma oncotic pressure, e.g. below 2 kPa (15 mmHg), decreases the gradient at the venous end of the capillary and consequently tissue fluid can then accumulate as oedema. Measurement of oncotic pressure may therefore help with the management of patients with pulmonary or tissue oedema. The instrument used for such measurements is an oncometer and is based on the principle shown in

Fig. 7.9. A semipermeable membrane separates the plasma sample from a saline reference solution, and the change due to oncotic pressure is measured by a transducer.

Osmolarity and Renal Function

In the kidney, filtrate passing from the glomerulus is concentrated by the cells in the renal tubules, as illustrated diagrammatically in Fig. 7.11. The plasma osmolarity is about 300 mosmol litre^{-1} and so the filtrate reaching the tubules is also close to this osmolarity. As the contribution of plasma proteins to the total osmolarity of plasma is very slight compared with that of the electrolytes, their absence from the filtrate is not an important factor. In the tubules, active reabsorption, especially of water, then takes place and the urine finally produced may have an osmolarity of about 1000 mosmol litre^{-1}, three to four times greater than the plasma osmolarity.

The relative osmolarity of the urine to that of the plasma gives a good index of the efficiency of renal function. If the urine osmolarity has fallen to that of the plasma, this suggests either that the patient is having a diuresis or that there is some impairment of renal function. In other words, a urine plasma osmolarity ratio of just over 1 with a low urine output suggests an impairment of renal tubular function.

In reports of urine osmolarity, an alternative expression, osmolality, is commonly used. Osmolality refers to the number of osmoles per kilogram of water or of other solvent. In scientific research, osmolality is the preferred term because it avoids inaccuracies from the effect of temperature on the volume of the solution. The analogous terms, molarity and molality, have a similar meaning of moles per litre of solution and moles per kilogram of water or other solvent, respectively.

Measurement of Osmolality

To measure the osmolality of urine or of plasma, an osmometer is used. Its principle is based on the depression of the freezing point of a solution, a phenomenon related to osmosis. This phenomenon is also the basis of the use of salt to melt ice on paths and roads. The depression of freezing point of a solution is directly proportional to its osmolality and 1 mol of a substance added to 1 kg of water depresses the freezing point by 1.86°C. Similarly, the depression of the freezing point of the water in plasma and urine is related to the osmolality and this principle is used in the osmometer, illustrated in Fig. 7.12.

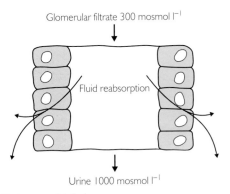

Glomerular filtrate 300 mosmol l^{-1}

Fluid reabsorption

Urine 1000 mosmol l^{-1}

Figure 7.11 Osmolarity in a renal tubule

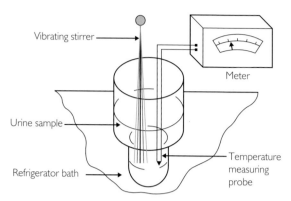

Figure 7.12 Osmometer based on the depression of the freezing point

Two millilitres of urine are put in the sample tube in the refrigerator bath and a measuring probe senses the temperature to give a reading on the meter. Initially, the temperature of the urine falls below its freezing point, a process known as supercooling, which occurs with some substances until freezing is initiated at some point in the liquid. Once freezing has started, it subsequently spreads throughout the fluid. In the osmometer, a vibrating stirrer is used to initiate freezing after supercooling has occurred. The sample then warms to a steady freezing point temperature as the solution changes state and this steady reading can be noted. To avoid the need to convert freezing point depression to milliosmoles, modern instruments are calibrated to give a direct indication of osmolality when the meter recording the temperature finally achieves a steady reading.

Depression of the freezing point is not the only effect of a dissolved substance. Figure 7.13 shows a pure solvent on the left and a solution with a solute present in the compartment on the right. Arrows above the liquid indicate that some solvent molecules vaporize to give rise to a vapour pressure above. On the right, the large solute molecules of the substance reduce the surface area available for the escape of the smaller solvent molecules. The solute therefore reduces the vapour pressure of the solvent. This effect is known as Raoult's law:

Raoult's law states that the depression or reduction of vapour pressure of a solvent is proportional to the molar concentration of the solute.

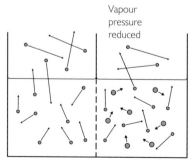

Figure 7.13 Illustration of Raoult's law

An osmometer using this principle of lowering of vapour pressure by a solute is also available. It has the advantage over osmometers which use the depression of freezing point in that it uses a smaller sample and can thus be used to measure the osmolality of sweat. The osmolality of sweat is proportional to its total electrolyte content, which is altered, for example, in patients suffering from cystic fibrosis.

A further effect caused by the presence of a solute in a solvent is a reduction in vapour pressure and a consequent increase in the boiling point.

The properties which depend on the osmolarity of a solution – i.e. osmotic pressure, freezing point depression, vapour pressure reduction and boiling point elevation – are sometimes known as the colligative properties of a solution.

Azeotropes

Raoult's law applies to all solutions and the substance dissolved in solution need not be a solid or a gas but may be another liquid. A special example of one liquid dissolved in another is an azeotrope.

An azeotrope is a mixture which vaporizes in the same proportions as the volume concentrations of the components in solution. Ether and halothane form an azeotrope, provided that they are in the ratio of one part of ether to two parts halothane by volume.

	Volume concentration	Mass concentration	Molar concentration
Ether	333 ml litre^{-1}	236 g litre^{-1}	3.19 mol litre^{-1}
Halothane	667 ml litre^{-1}	1240 g litre^{-1}	6.30 mol litre^{-1}

By application of the density and the molecular weights of ether and halothane, respectively, the mass concentrations and molar concentrations may be calculated. As shown in the table, the ratio of the molar concentrations is 1 to 2 and so, by Raoult's law, the vapour pressure will also be in this same proportion. This means that the components of this azeotrope evaporate in the ratio of one part of ether to two parts of halothane, so the relative volume concentrations of the liquid mixture do not change. Azeotropes are found for other mixtures; thus alcohol and water form an azeotrope in the proportions of 96% alcohol and 4% water. This means that the components of this azeotrope evaporate in the ratio of 96 parts of alcohol to 4 parts of water, thus making it impossible to reduce the concentration of water in the mixture further by fractional distillation.

Work, Energy and Power

8

Work

This chapter concentrates on work, energy and power, with special reference to ventilation and cardiac output. Mechanical work is a form of energy, and other forms of energy include heat energy and chemical energy. Work is done or energy is expended whenever the point of application of a force moves in the direction of the force. The SI unit of energy is the joule:

One joule of work is done when a force of one newton moves its point of application one metre in the direction of the force.

The force of gravity on an apple which has a mass of 102 grams is 1 newton, so if the apple is raised 1 metre vertically against the force of gravity, 1 joule of work is performed, as illustrated in Fig. 8.1. The total energy must remain constant and, in this case, the mechanical energy expended in raising the apple is converted into potential energy represented by the additional height of the apple.

Forces in the body normally arise from muscular contraction; the shortening of the muscle multiplied by the mean force exerted is the mechanical work performed.

Work of a Ventilator During Inspiration

A constant-pressure generator type of ventilator (Fig. 8.2) gives a good example of the interrelationship between the force and distance moved, and the pressure and volume changes. In this example, the force of gravity F on mass M acts over the area A to give a pressure P. During the descent of the bellows through a distance D, a volume of air V is delivered.

Work done = $F \times D$

Figure 8.1 Illustration of the definition of the joule

⊢ 1 metre

1 newton

Figure 8.2 Work of inspiration for a perfect constant-pressure generator ventilator

but

$$P = \frac{F}{A} \text{ therefore } F = PA$$

and

$$V = D \times A \text{ therefore } D = \frac{V}{A}$$

Consequently,

$$\text{Work done} = PA \times \frac{V}{A} = PV$$

It can be seen that the work done is the product of the volume of gas moved and the pressure required.

Figure 8.2 also shows the volume–pressure graph of the inspiration, and the shaded rectangular area equals PV or the work done by the perfect constant-pressure generator ventilator in one inspiration. In this example the pressure from the ventilator increases rapidly to 0.6 kPa (6 cmH$_2$O) above atmospheric pressure and remains steady at this value until the lungs are inflated with 0.5 litre of air. The work done by the ventilator can be calculated in SI units, provided that pressure is expressed in pascals and volume in cubic metres (1 m^3 = 10^3 litres):

$$\text{Work done} = (0.6 \times 10^3) \text{ Pa} \times (0.5 \times 10^{-3}) \text{ m}^3$$

$$= 0.3 \text{ J}$$

$$= 300 \text{ mJ}$$

Thus, this inspiration requires 300 mJ of work.

During expiration, the pressure at the ventilator falls rapidly to atmospheric pressure and remains at zero while the air is expired. The dotted line on the graph (Fig. 8.2) shows the pressure and volume changes during expiration.

For simplification, a constant-pressure generator has been chosen for this example, but few ventilators act as perfect constant-pressure generators.

Most ventilators give a smoother build-up of pressure, as indicated in Fig. 8.3, but the concept that the shaded area enclosed by the loop indicates the work of the ventilator for one inspiration is still valid. In this case, the calculation of the area is more complex and uses the process of integration (considered in Chapter 25).

Energy Changes

Energy cannot be lost but is converted from one form to another. During inspiration, about half the mechanical energy used is stored as potential energy in the

Figure 8.3
Volume–pressure graph for inspiration and expiration with a typical ventilator

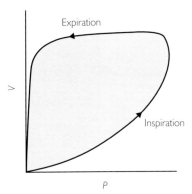

elastic tissues of the lung and the chest wall. This energy is subsequently used for the work of expiration. The remaining half of the mechanical energy of inspiration is used in overcoming airway resistance and in moving the air and tissues.

Figure 8.4 illustrates a model to help understand the energy changes during inspiration. A ventilator of a constant-pressure generator type is attached to the patient via a cycling device. The patient's lungs are represented by a syringe in which movement of the plunger is opposed by the stretching of an elastic band. In this model the plunger represents the diaphragm and the elastic band represents the elasticity of the lung tissues and chest wall. The resistance to the flow of air into the syringe represents the airway resistance and the pressure within the syringe is indicated by P_L. It is assumed that the end-inspiratory pressure in the syringe reaches the pressure P_M provided by the ventilator.

As previously explained, the total work done by the constant-pressure generator ventilator for one inspiration is represented by the rectangular area PV in the graph (Fig. 8.5). This energy can be divided into two parts: energy used in stretching the elastic band and energy used in overcoming resistance to airflow into the syringe.

To assess the energy used in stretching the elastic band, consider how the pressure P_L changes within the syringe. This could represent the pressure changes within the alveoli. At the start of inspiration, the elastic band is unstretched, so the pressure in the syringe is atmospheric pressure. The pressure in the syringe increases linearly with volume as air flows into the syringe, tracing the line C–D

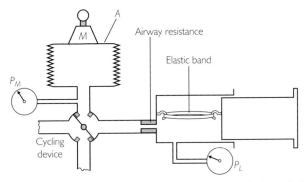

Figure 8.4 Simple syringe model to illustrate inspiration in controlled ventilation; an elastic band represents the elasticity of the lung and chest wall

Figure 8.5 Graph of pressure change P_L in the model lung syringe during inflation with a volume of 0.5 litre; the ventilator pressure P_M is also indicated

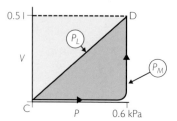

on the graph, the slope of which represents compliance. The average pressure is half the end-inspiratory pressure P, so the work done against the elastic band is $\frac{1}{2}PV$ and is equal to the area of the shaded section of the volume–pressure graph bounded by the line C–D.

The difference between this area and the total area PV is shown in the stippled section of the volume–pressure graph and represents the energy expended in moving the gas against the airway resistance. In the example at the start of inspiration, P_L is zero, as the syringe has been open to atmospheric pressure, and the ventilator pressure P_M is 0.6 kPa, so the initial pressure gradient across the airway resistance is 0.6 kPa. This gradient decreases to zero at the end of inspiration and so the average pressure difference is again $\frac{1}{2}P$ and the energy expended in moving the gas is $\frac{1}{2}PV$.

Work of Expiration

The syringe model (Fig. 8.4) may also be used to illustrate expiration. The cycling device is open to the atmosphere and the pressure within the syringe then falls linearly to zero if plotted against the volume expired. The work expended is consequently $\frac{1}{2}PV$ and is used in overcoming the airway resistance in the model. In patients, the tissue resistance of the lungs and chest wall is present in addition to airway resistance, but is not illustrated in the model.

Work of Inspiration in Spontaneous Breathing

In a quiet inspiration the contraction of the diaphragm muscle draws down the diaphragm by about 15 mm, causing a reduction of pressure within the chest and the inspiration of air. To represent this, the syringe model must be modified to that shown in Fig. 8.6. The syringe now has two plungers with fluid between them. The fluid represents the thin layer of serous fluid in the intrapleural space, whereas the right-hand plunger represents the diaphragm and the left-hand plunger represents the lung tissues moved.

The pressure in the intrapleural space is subatmospheric due to the elasticity of the band and decreases further as a result of the contraction of the diaphragm, represented by the force shown on the right-hand plunger. Through the fluid coupling of the intrapleural space, this force is transferred to the lungs and inspiration occurs. A plot of volume against intrapleural pressure for a typical inspiration is shown in Fig. 8.6. As in the case of controlled ventilation, the stippled area on the graph gives the work expended in overcoming airway resistance and the triangular shaded area gives the stored elastic energy which is used during expiration.

If in this model 0.5 litre of air is inspired when the average pressure in the coupling fluid is 0.6 kPa, then 300 mJ of work is done in inspiration.

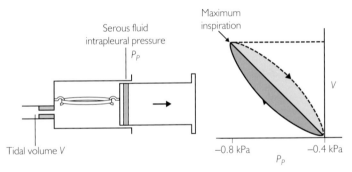

Figure 8.6 Model illustrating spontaneous inspiration: the space between the two plungers represents the intrapleural space

This simple syringe model does not show the chest expansion which also occurs, and which accounts for 10–40% of the inspired tidal volume. This expansion is caused by three factors: the diaphragm acting on the lower margin of the rib cage to raise it, the intercostal muscles, especially the external intercostals, acting to raise the ribs, and the scalene muscles raising the upper ribs of the thoracic cage.

The initial energy for the contraction of the inspiratory muscles originates in the high-energy bonds of adenosine triphosphate (ATP) and most of this energy has in turn arisen from that released during the combination of oxygen with water and electrons in the respiratory chains of enzymes:

$$O_2 + 2H_2O + 4e = 4OH^- + Energy$$

In the respiratory muscles, 10% of the chemical energy is turned into mechanical energy and 90% into heat. Figure 8.7 summarizes the energy changes for a typical inspiration and expiration.

Measuring the Work of Inspiration

In controlled ventilation, analysis of a graph of airway pressure against volume change gives the work of inspiration, but the total work of inspiration is more

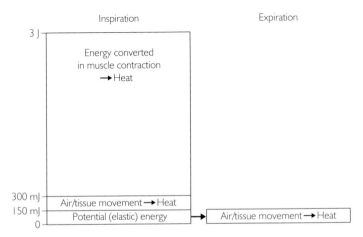

Figure 8.7 Energy changes during inspiration and expiration

difficult to measure in a spontaneously breathing patient. Although the volume inspired may be measured by a pneumotachograph (Chapter 3), the pressures exerted by the respiratory muscles in the chest wall cannot be monitored directly. Intrapleural pressure changes, however, indicate pressure changes acting on the lung, and the pressure in the lower oesophagus can be measured by a catheter with a balloon at its tip and used as an indication of these pressure changes.

Figure 8.6 illustrates the graph of volume against pressure which might be obtained in this way, but in this example the resistive and elastic work against the tissues of the chest wall are not measured. During expiration, the graph traces the curve shown by the dotted line. The greater the expiratory resistance, the greater the bowing of this line to the right; the medium-shaded area to the left of this dotted line represents the expiratory work done against airway and lung tissue resistance, whereas the balance of the stored energy in the triangular area is converted into heat in the tissues.

This technique has its limitations; not only does it exclude the work of movement of the chest wall but also the oesophageal pressure readings cannot give absolute accuracy. This is because they can indicate pleural pressure at only one site and the pleural pressure varies according to both the site of measurement and the posture of the patient.

Power of Breathing

Power is the rate of working and is measured in watts. 1 watt is 1 joule per second:

$$W = J \ s^{-1}$$

In the earlier example, the work of one inspiration was 300 mJ. If the respiration rate is 16 per minute, the power of breathing is calculated as follows:

$$\text{Mechanical power of breathing} = 300 \ mJ \times \frac{16}{60} \ s^{-1} = 80 \ mW$$

Efficiency of Respiratory Muscles

The respiratory muscles are only 10% efficient in producing mechanical energy, the rest of the energy being dissipated as heat. Thus, the actual energy requirements in the example above would be 10 times greater than 80 mW, i.e. about 800 mW. As the normal metabolic rate is about 80 W under resting conditions (Chapter 9), in this example the energy requirements for breathing would be 1% of the total metabolism.

Effect of Type of Flow

The power of breathing depends on the type of flow in the air passages, as pressure gradients are greater when the flow is turbulent than when it is laminar (Chapter 2). Consider, for example, the energy used as fluid flows through a tube. As the product of average pressure difference and volume moved indicates the energy, pressure difference across a tube multiplied by the fluid flow gives the power, if the pressure difference is small compared with atmospheric pressure.

Energy $E = P \times V$

Therefore

Power $\dot{E} = P \times \dot{V}$

In the case of laminar flow, pressure is proportional to flow:

$$P_L \propto \dot{V}_L$$

Therefore

Power in laminar flow $\dot{E}_L \propto \dot{V}_L{}^2$

In the case of turbulent flow, pressure is proportional to the square of the flow:

$$PT \propto \dot{V}_L{}^2$$

Therefore

Power in turbulent flow $E_T \propto \dot{V}_T{}^3$

It is seen that the power dissipated as fluid flows through a tube varies between the square and the cube of the flow.

The above calculations are simplified in that they do not allow for the kinetic energy in the flowing fluid, but in the flow normally present in the respiratory and circulatory systems the kinetic energy is very small.

Effect of Hyperventilation in Patients

In quiet ventilation, flow is predominantly laminar but becomes turbulent as ventilation increases, so that during hyperventilation the power of breathing increases rapidly at a rate approaching the cube of the gas flow. As the gas flow in the airway is more or less proportional to the tidal ventilation, the power of breathing increases rapidly with hyperventilation at a rate approaching the cube of the tidal ventilation, and a high oxygen consumption by the respiratory muscles occurs.

In some respiratory diseases the oxygen requirements of the respiratory muscles during hyperventilation become considerable and exceed the extra oxygen which is transported by the increased ventilation. Hence, pharmacological stimulation of ventilation in respiratory disease carries the risk of hypoxia in such patients.

Lung Compliance and Airway Resistance

Detailed consideration of these factors is beyond the scope of this book, but it should be noted that the power of respiration varies with the respiratory rate and that for a given patient there is an optimum respiratory rate depending on the compliance of the lungs and on airway resistance.

The time constant for the lungs is the product of compliance and resistance (Chapter 5). Patients with a low time constant tend to have a rapid respiratory rate whereas a high time constant is associated with a slower rate.

Work of Myocardial Contraction

The area of a graph of the changes in cardiac pressure and volume can be used to measure the work of myocardial contraction in the same way that the area of a pressure–volume loop in ventilation can be used to indicate the energy changes in breathing.

Figure 8.8 shows a tracing of the volume and pressure changes in the left ventricle during a typical cardiac cycle. The pressure and volume axes are reversed from those given when ventilation was discussed, as this is the more usual presentation when considering cardiac physiology. In this example, the left ventricular volume increased 60 ml during diastolic filling, then the pressure increased from

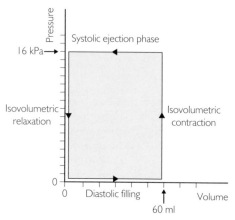

Figure 8.8 Volume and pressure in the left ventricle during a typical cardiac cycle

0 to 16 kPa (0–120 mmHg) during isovolumetric contraction. The systolic ejection phase and isovolumetric relaxation are indicated on Fig. 8.8, and the area of the loop represents the work done.

$$\text{Work done} = (16 \times 10^3) \text{ Pa} \times (60 \times 10^{-6}) \text{ m}^3$$

$$= 960 \times 10^{-3} \text{ J}$$

$$= 960 \text{ mJ}$$

Thus one myocardial contraction of the left ventricle requires just under 1 joule of work. If the heart rate is 60, then the power of the left ventricle of the heart is about 60 joules per minute, i.e. 1 watt.

To make such measurements of work, a continuous ventricular pressure recording may be obtained from an intraventricular cardiac catheter, and volume measurements may be deduced from ultrasonic flow measurement (Chapter 13) or estimated from echocardiography (Chapter 13), cineangiography or other imaging techniques.

Power of the Heart

The concept of power as a product of pressure difference and fluid flow may also be applied to the cardiac output. For example, if the mean arterial pressure is 12 kPa (90 mmHg), the pulmonary venous pressure 0 kPa and the left cardiac output 5 litres min^{-1}, then the power of the left heart can be calculated from the product of the pressure and flow:

$$\dot{E} = P \times \dot{V}$$

$$\text{Power of left heart} = 12 \times 10^3 \text{ Pa} \times \frac{5 \times 10^{-3}}{60} \text{ m}^3 \text{ s}^{-1} = 1 \text{ W}$$

The power of the right heart can be similarly calculated as follows. If the mean pulmonary artery pressure is 2.4 kPa (18 mmHg) above the central venous pressure, then:

$$\text{Power of right heart} = 2.4 \times 10^3 \text{ Pa} \times \frac{5 \times 10^{-3}}{60} \text{ m}^3 \text{ s}^{-1} = 0.2 \text{ W}$$

Total power of heart = 1.2 W

If the efficiency of the heart were 15% in this instance, then the total energy requirements of 8 W would be 10% of a typical basal metabolism of 80 W.

Energy is also generated by the heart to provide the kinetic energy of the flowing blood, but this is a relatively small component of the total power.

To make the measurements for the above example the mean arterial pressure could be obtained from an arterial pressure trace and pulmonary pressures from cardiac catheterization, whereas cardiac output could be measured by a thermal dilution technique (Chapter 5) or by a technique based upon the Fick principle (Chapter 3).

Effect of Blood Pressure and Cardiac Output on the Work of the Heart

As power is the product of pressure and flow, the work of the heart is directly proportional to the mean blood pressure and to the cardiac output.

Hypertension results in additional energy requirements even if the cardiac output is unchanged, and hypotension lowers the energy demands on the heart provided that cardiac output is not simultaneously raised. A high cardiac output due to any cause (e.g. thyrotoxicosis, anaemia or exercise) also increases the work load of the heart. An increase in the energy requirements of the heart, if maintained, may lead to heart failure.

Temperature

The Concept of Temperature and Heat

Heat is a form of energy that can be transferred from a hotter substance to a colder substance, the energy being in the form of the kinetic energy of the molecules of the substance. Temperature is the thermal state of a substance which determines whether it will give heat to another substance or receive heat from it, heat being transferred from the substance at the higher temperature to the substance at the lower temperature. As described in Chapter 4, the temperature of a gas is a measure of the speed at which the molecules are moving.

An analogy may be drawn between the relationship of heat to temperature and the relationship of the quantity of a solute to its concentration. Thus, in the same way that temperature rises as heat energy is added to a substance, so concentration rises as a solute is added to a solution. In each case, if the substance or solution is divided into two equal parts, each part will have the same temperature or concentration although the heat energy or quantity of solute in each case is halved.

Temperature Scales

When heat energy is added to a substance, not only does its temperature rise but also changes in its physical properties occur. For example, the substance may expand, and its electrical resistance may change. Use is made of such phenomena in temperature measurement and in the construction of temperature scales. Thus, mercury, which expands and contracts as the temperature changes, was the substance used by Fahrenheit to construct the first temperature scale.

Normally, temperature scales have arbitrarily chosen fixed points, one example of which is the triple point of water, the temperature at which ice, water and water vapour are all in equilibrium.

In the SI system, the unit of temperature is the kelvin, which is defined as the fraction 1/273.16 of the thermodynamic temperature of the triple point of water. The Celsius scale is also approved and the intervals on this scale are identical to those on the kelvin scale (K), but the relationship between the two is as follows:

Temperature (K) = Temperature (°C) + 273.15

Thus, on the Celsius scale, the triple point of water occurs at a temperature of 0.01°C. Note also that the degree symbol (°) is not used with the kelvin symbol (K).

Non-Electrical Techniques of Temperature Measurement

The mercury thermometer, which utilizes the change in volume of mercury with temperature, is a reliable system, used both in laboratories and in hospital wards.

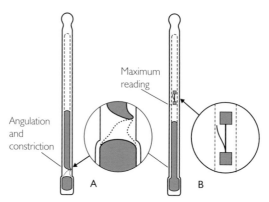

Figure 9.1 Maximum reading thermometers

An advantage in clinical use is that it can be made in maximum reading form, achieved by an angled constriction at the lower part of the mercury column which splits the mercury column after it has reached its maximum reading (Fig. 9.1A). This prevents the mercury above from contracting into the bulb until the thermometer is shaken.

Maximum reading thermometers may also be made by including a small metal index above the surface of the mercury, as shown in Fig. 9.1B. When the mercury column contracts, this index is left behind at the level of maximum temperature.

The mercury thermometer has two main disadvantages in clinical practice: first, 2–3 min are necessary for complete thermal equilibrium between the mercury and its surroundings; and, secondly, it may be difficult to introduce the thermometer into some orifices because of its rigidity and the risk of its breaking, with consequent injury to the patient.

Alcohol is sometimes used instead of mercury in thermometers. It is cheaper and is more suitable for use at very low temperatures, because mercury solidifies at −39°C. On the other hand, these thermometers are unsuitable for high temperatures, because alcohol boils at 78.5°C.

Dial thermometers may use either a bimetallic strip or a Bourdon gauge. Figure 9.2 shows a bimetallic strip thermometer, the sensing element of which consists of two dissimilar metals fixed together in a coil. As the temperature rises, the

Figure 9.2 Bimetallic strip thermometer

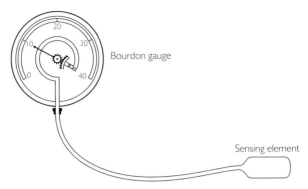

Figure 9.3 Bourdon gauge thermometer

metals expand by different amounts and the coil tightens to move the lever clockwise over the scale.

The Bourdon gauge type of thermometer is shown in Fig. 9.3. This gauge is really a device for measuring pressure, and is attached to a sensing element containing a small tube of mercury or a volatile fluid. Variation in temperature causes a volume or pressure change in the sensing fluid and this is recorded on the Bourdon gauge, which is calibrated in units of temperature.

Electrical Techniques of Temperature Measurement

There are three principal electrical techniques for measuring temperature: the resistance thermometer, the thermistor and the thermocouple.

The resistance thermometer is based on the fact that the electrical resistance of a metal increases linearly with temperature. A simple resistance thermometer could incorporate a platinum wire resistor, a battery as a source of electrical potential and an ammeter to measure current, which could then be calibrated to indicate temperature. Unfortunately, a simple system of this type would not be very sensitive and it is better to incorporate the temperature-sensitive resistor into a Wheatstone bridge circuit containing an array of resistors. This circuit is dealt with in Chapter 14.

Another electrical temperature system is based on the use of a thermistor. The usual type of thermistor is a small bead of metal oxide, the resistance of which – unlike the platinum resistance thermometer – falls exponentially as the temperature rises (Fig. 9.4). Special thermistors, however, are also available in which

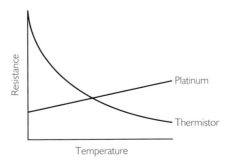

Figure 9.4 The changes of resistance with temperature for a platinum resistance thermometer and a thermistor

resistance rises with temperature. In the clinical temperature range, the thermistor undergoes greater resistance change than the platinum resistance thermometer and, as with the latter, it is often used in a Wheatstone bridge circuit. The thermistor has the added advantage that the metal oxide bead can be made very small and that it can be manufactured more cheaply than the platinum resistance thermometer. A disadvantage is that the calibration is liable to change if the thermistor is subjected to severe changes of temperature, e.g. during heat sterilization.

Another system of measuring temperature is based on the Seebeck effect; the principle is shown in Fig. 9.5. At any junction of two dissimilar metals a small voltage is produced, the magnitude of which depends on the temperature of the junction. A junction of this type is known as a thermocouple, and metals such as copper and constantan may be used; constantan is an alloy of copper and nickel. A second junction is needed to form a complete electric circuit, but at this junction another temperature-dependent voltage will develop. For the thermocouple to be used as a thermometer, one of the junctions, the reference junction, must be kept at a constant temperature while the measuring junction acts as a temperature probe; alternatively, the equipment may provide electrical compensation for changes in reference junction temperature. An advantage of the thermocouple is that the measuring probe can be manufactured and used in the form of a needle.

The response time of temperature measuring probes which use electrical effects depends mostly on size and may range from 0.1 s to 15 s. Small probes have a smaller heat capacity (Chapter 10) than large probes and therefore a shorter response time. A fast response is important for thermistors used for the measurement of cardiac output by the thermal dilution technique (Chapter 5).

Infrared Ear and Tympanic Membrane Thermometers

Infrared ear and tympanic membrane thermometers are based on the fact that objects emit electromagnetic radiation over a range of wavelengths. The intensity of this radiation and the wavelength for which the intensity of emitted radiation is a maximum depend on the temperature of the object. Objects at body temperature primarily emit infrared radiation. The infrared ear thermometer uses a tube inserted into the ear canal to direct the radiation emitted by the ear drum and ear canal on to a sensor which converts the radiation into an electrical signal. Tympanic membrane thermometers are intended to be inserted further into the ear so that they receive radiation only from the tympanic membrane, the temperature

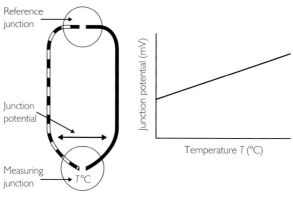

Figure 9.5 Seebeck effect; principle of the thermocouple

of which is more representative of core temperature than the ear canal. Two types of sensor are in use.

The pyroelectric sensor is made of a type of ceramic crystalline material in which the electric charges on the molecules are slightly separated, a property known as polarization. If the temperature of such a material is altered – for example, by incident radiation – the polarization changes. This change in polarization can be detected as an electrical signal if electrodes are placed on opposite faces of a thin slice of the material to form a capacitor. When the polarization changes, the movement of charge appears as a voltage between the electrodes on either side of the slice. The sensor will only produce an electrical output signal when the temperature changes: i.e. when the level of incident radiation changes. The electrical signal is proportional to the magnitude and rate of change of the temperature difference across the capacitor. Infrared thermometers using pyroelectric sensors therefore employ a shutter mechanism to provide a controlled period of exposure to the infrared radiation.

The thermopile sensor is constructed of many thermocouples connected in parallel. It allows continuous readings.

Because infrared thermometers determine the temperature of infrared emission from a source, rather than absorbing heat from the object and coming into thermal equilibrium with it, they have a short response time, typically less than 5 s.

Clinical Applications

There is a choice of many sites for temperature measurement in patients: for example, the mercury clinical thermometer may be used in the mouth, axilla or rectum, but there is a limitation to its use owing to its rigidity. Rectal temperature measurement is of less value than measurements from other sites because, apart from aesthetic considerations, there is a risk in small babies of perforation of the rectum, whereas in adults rectal temperature measurements may be inaccurate owing to the slowness with which rectal temperature equilibrates with body temperature.

The measuring probes of electrical thermometers may be introduced into other sites such as the nose, ear or oesophagus and they may also be applied to the skin. One popular site is the lower oesophagus; in this case it is important that the recording tip of the thermometer is not too high, because the temperature of the oesophagus may then be reduced owing to the proximity of the lower trachea, which is cooled by inspired air. The ear may also been used as a site to measure body temperature, but the obvious drawback to this site is the risk of perforation of the drum.

Nasal temperature fluctuates widely because of the passage of inspired and expired air and this fact has been utilized in the design of respiratory monitors, as illustrated on the left of Fig. 9.6. The pulses from fluctuation of temperature over the thermistor bead are electronically processed to give the respiration rate. The nose may be used as an alternative to the oesophagus to measure body temperature in an anaesthetized patient intubated with a cuffed endotracheal tube – as shown on the right of the figure – because there is then no respiratory air movement to cool the nasal cavity.

Skin temperature measurements are useful in anaesthesia because a fall of skin temperature in the periphery can be correlated with the degree of shock in an ill patient.

A special system for measuring skin temperature is called thermography. In this technique, the radiant heat from the patient's skin is imaged by means of an

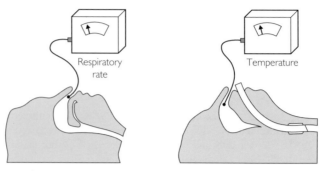

Figure 9.6 Use of nasal temperature to monitor respiratory rate or body temperature

infrared-sensitive camera to provide a thermograph of the relative warmth of the skin. Different colours in the thermograph indicate temperature differences and these, in turn, give an indication of the underlying vascularity. In this way, thermography has been used to detect tumours and vascular abnormalities.

Body Temperature

Humans, like all mammals and birds, are homeothermic and control their central body temperature within a narrow range despite a wide range of environmental temperature. In man, this range is normally $37 \pm 0.5°C$. A constant temperature is essential, as variation in temperature may bring about changes in enzyme reaction rates governing physiological processes and some metabolic processes could not occur if body temperature were allowed to cool to that of the environment.

Slight variation in body temperature, however, does occur naturally in man. There is a circadian or diurnal rhythm of around 0.4°C, the temperature being lowest in the early morning and reaching a maximum in the early evening. There is also a slight variation in body temperature during the menstrual cycle in women, with the basal temperature rising after ovulation for the second half of the cycle. Exercise can also cause a rise in body temperature; this increase may be as much as 2°C if energy expenditure is large.

As shown in Fig. 9.7, it is the central core of the body which is maintained at the constant temperature; the surface layer or shell of the body is at a lower, more

Figure 9.7 Core and shell temperatures in the body; the intermediate zone represents variable core size

variable temperature, which can range from 32 to 35°C, depending on physiological factors. The central core includes the brain, thoracic and abdominal organs and also some of the deep tissues of the limbs, the amount varying with the environmental temperature as represented by the intermediate zone. The shell is a layer with a variable depth of around 2.5 cm. The temperature in the body core depends on the balance between heat production in the core and heat loss through the shell or surface layer.

The difference between core temperature and average skin temperature is thus a useful measurement.

Heat Production

Heat production is determined by the general metabolic rate of the person at any given time and is measured in watts. In an average man under resting conditions, heat production is of the order of 50 W m^{-2} body surface area or 80 W total, but increases of metabolic rate occur because of food consumption, exercise and other factors. In addition, an increase in metabolic rate is found when there is a rise of body temperature. There is no mechanism by which heat production can be reduced to compensate for overheating, but an increase of heat production can be provided by shivering.

Minor shivering is not apparent to the naked eye and may be detected only by an electromyogram. Major shivering is needed only when a large increase in heat production is required. Such shivering can more than double the metabolic heat production and a fivefold increase is possible in special circumstances. The onset of shivering does not normally occur until the body's mechanisms for the control of heat loss have already been activated.

Heat Loss

There are four principal routes of heat loss from the body: radiation, convection, evaporation of water and heat loss through respiration. Although the relative importance of these routes varies with the environment, their typical contributions to the total heat loss are given in Table 9.1.

Conduction from one solid body to another is not important per se as a route of heat loss from the body. Conduction is the process whereby heat energy is transmitted through a substance by the transfer of the energy of motion of the molecules to adjacent molecules. Metals and some crystals are good conductors of heat but gases are poor conductors, and the air surrounding an individual provides protection from heat loss through conduction unless excess air movement is present.

Heat loss from radiation is important and may account for up to 50% of normal heat loss from the body. A hot object emits radiation over a spectrum of wavelengths predominantly in the infrared region. The radiation emitted carries energy

Table 9.1 Contributions to the heat loss

Type of radiation	Approximate contribution to heat loss
Radiation	40%
Convection	30%
Evaporation	20%
Respiration	10% (8% evaporation of water; 2% heating of air)

from the hot object, thus causing it to cool down. Conversely, if this radiation is absorbed by another object, that object will become hotter. Thus radiation can transfer heat energy between two objects which are not in contact, the rate of transfer depending on the relative temperatures and the surface characteristics of the objects. Radiant heat losses are increased if the body is surrounded by cold objects and reduced by radiation received from warm surroundings. Space blankets of shiny reflective metallized plastic foil are sometimes used to restrict radiant heat loss, but should not be used in theatre areas because of the increased risks of burns and of electric shock (Chapter 16). Metallized reflective caps have, however, come into use, as heat loss from the head can be considerable.

Convection is an important route of heat loss. In convection, the air layer adjacent to the surface of the body is warmed by conduction and, as it is heated, it expands and becomes less dense and so rises. The resulting convection current carries heat away from the subject.

Surface evaporative heat loss is due to the loss of latent heat of vaporization of moisture on the skin's surface (Chapter 10). The loss of heat by this route is dependent on the water vapour pressure gradient from the skin to the air and on the total area of moist skin exposed to the atmosphere. The amount of heat lost by this route may be increased 10-fold by sweating, which increases the amount of moisture available for evaporation on the skin surface.

All these routes of heat loss depend on the total area of skin exposed to the environment. Consequently, if this area is reduced, heat loss is diminished. The rate of heat loss is also influenced by insulation, which constitutes a resistance to heat loss and arises from several sources. The body tissues lying between the core and the skin surface consist mainly of fat, which forms a relatively avascular insulating layer. Clothing, too, acts not only by reducing the amount of skin surface area exposed but also by trapping air. So the trapped air, a poor conductor of heat, acts as an insulator.

Respiration accounts for only a small amount of the total heat loss, typically perhaps 10%. Eight per cent of this loss occurs through increasing the humidity of the inspired air from about 50% to 100%, and 2% is due to warming the air. In humans, this route of heat loss is not an important mechanism for the physiological control of temperature, but changes in respiratory heat loss occur in anaesthesia. For example, inspiration of dry gases increases the heat lost through respiration and may contribute to the risk of hypothermia as explained in Chapter 10.

Responses to Changes in Environmental Temperature

Physiological control over temperature is mediated by temperature receptors in the skin and by a temperature receptor in the hypothalamus which is sensitive to the temperature of the blood perfusing it. Both types of sensor signal to a thermoregulatory centre in the hypothalamus and so initiate appropriate reflex changes. In the case of mild changes of environmental temperature, reflex changes of vascular tone occur and these alter skin temperature and so alter heat loss. In the case of major cooling of the body, reflexes elicit shivering, whereas excessive heat causes reflex sweating and vasodilation. Signals from the thermoregulatory centre to the cerebral cortex lead to appropriate behavioural responses, so that the person concerned can alter the amount of clothing or the level of activity.

Hypothermia

The thermoregulatory centre is depressed by anaesthesia and many anaesthetics also have an effect on vasomotor tone, giving peripheral vasodilation and thus increased heat loss. During surgery there is a greater area of the patient exposed to the atmosphere, in addition to which the loss of heat may be increased by rapid air movement from modern theatre ventilation. A patient's temperature may also be reduced as a result of the intravenous infusion of cold fluids.

In prolonged surgery. therefore, there is a risk of hypothermia and the patient's core temperature must be monitored and appropriate measures taken to maintain it. Such measures include raising theatre temperature, using a forced air warmer, heating and humidifying inspired gases and warming infused fluids.

Hypothermia may be induced intentionally in anaesthetized patients undergoing neurosurgery or cardiac surgery. The reduced body temperature decreases metabolism and thus the tissue demand for oxygen, so that blood flow to vital areas may be interrupted for a time without the risk of hypoxic damage. Thus at 30°C, the time for safe circulatory occlusion is double that at 37°C. In the simpler hypothermic techniques, core temperatures of below 30°C are avoided because otherwise there is a risk of ventricular fibrillation, but lower temperatures are sometimes used in patients on extracorporeal circulation.

Pyrexia

In fever, the thermostat of the thermoregulatory centre may be regarded as being set at a higher level than normal, and this is usually due to a bacterial or endogenous pyrogen. Temperatures over 42°C cause cerebral impairment and disturbance of the physiological control mechanisms of heat loss by sweating. At high body temperatures over 45°C, the rise of temperature induces a rise in metabolism which leads to a vicious circle with even more heat being produced; the outcome is usually fatal. A problem at these high body temperatures is that heat production rises exponentially with temperature while the heat loss rises at a slower rate. Consequently, a temperature is reached above which heat production exceeds the maximum heat loss and the temperature then rises until death occurs.

A rare anaesthetic cause of such hyperpyrexia is the malignant hyperpyrexia which occurs in susceptible patients who have an abnormal response to volatile anaesthetic agents or suxamethonium. The condition is genetically determined and is associated with a dramatic rise in body temperature due to a massive increase in heat production, carrying a serious risk of fatality if not treated correctly.

Thermal Burns

There is a risk of burns and tissue damage if the temperature of the surface skin or tissues approaches 45°C from an external heat source. The actual temperature reached depends on the rate at which heat arrives from the heat source and the rate at which it is removed by the blood flow; consequently, burns are more likely in patients who are vasoconstricted or shocked. Examples of external heat sources are lamps, electric blankets and heated water-filled mattresses. Electrical burns are considered in Chapter 14 and the danger from fires in Chapter 23.

Heat Capacity and Latent Heat

10

The relationship between heat and temperature is considered in Chapter 9. When heat is applied to a substance, its temperature rises and, conversely, when heat is removed from a substance, its temperature falls. The quantity of heat necessary to produce a given change in temperature depends on the specific heat capacity of a substance:

Specific heat capacity is defined as the amount of heat required to raise the temperature of 1 kilogram of a substance by 1 kelvin (SI unit of specific heat capacity $J\ kg^{-1}\ K^{-1}$).

As 1 K is commensurate with 1°C, the specific heat capacity is often quoted using the latter unit. The word 'specific' in a definition indicates that the quantity is expressed in terms of unit mass. Specific heat capacity is often abbreviated to specific heat and must not be confused with the term 'heat capacity':

Heat capacity is defined as the amount of heat required to raise the temperature of a given object by 1 kelvin (SI unit of heat capacity $J\ K^{-1}$).

It is seen that heat capacity applies to an object or substance as a whole; consequently, it can be calculated from the product of the specific heat capacity and the mass. An example of heat capacity is given in Chapter 11 when vaporizers are considered. If an object such as a vaporizer has several component parts of different materials, its heat capacity can be calculated by adding the capacities of the components. In the case of a person, the tissue specific heat capacities can be approximated to a mean value of 3.5 kJ kg^{-1} °C^{-1} and the product of this and the patient's weight indicates the total heat capacity. For a 70 kg patient it would be 245 kJ °C^{-1}.

Knowledge of the heat capacity facilitates calculation of the effect of changes in heat production. Consider, for example, a patient after anaesthesia whose body temperature has fallen to 36°C. By shivering, the patient may increase heat production fourfold to 320 W from a basal level of 80 W. This is an extra 240 W or 240×60 joules per minute, i.e. 14.4 kJ min^{-1}. As 245 kJ are needed to raise the temperature one degree, this patient will need to shiver for 17 min to produce the heat required to do this.

The concept of body heat content has been used to estimate the overall heat gain or heat loss of a person or an object. The body heat content is the product of mean temperature and heat capacity. In the case of a person there are temperature gradients between the core and the shell; consequently, both core temperatures and surface skin temperatures must be measured and a mean body temperature calculated allowing for estimated sizes of core and shell tissues.

Figure 10.1 Specific heat of water

The term 'thermal capacity' is also sometimes encountered, but is best avoided because it may mean either specific heat or heat capacity.

As shown in Fig. 10.1, 4.18 kJ are required to raise the temperature of 1 kg of water by 1°C. The specific heat of water is therefore 4.18 kJ kg^{-1} °C^{-1}. In parenteral nutrition studies, however, calories and kilocalories may be used, 1 calorie being equal to 4.18 joules; so the specific heat of water is 1 kcal kg^{-1} °C^{-1}. It should be noted that in dietetics, the kilocalorie is often written as Calorie with a capital C.

The specific heat of most other substances is less than that of water. The high specific heat of water is used in the design of some vaporizers to provide a reservoir of heat and so maintain a steadier temperature. Thus, on older anaesthetic machines, a water reservoir was sometimes used around the Boyle's bottle vaporizer.

The high specific heat of cold infusion liquids and blood used in transfusions increases the cooling effect in the patient. The specific heat capacity of blood is 3.6 kJ kg^{-1} °C^{-1}.

Suppose 2 kg of blood, approximately 2 litres, are transfused at 5°C and warmed up to 35°C in the patient.

Heat required = 2 kg × 3.6 kJ kg^{-1} °C^{-1} × (35 − 5)°C

= (2 × 3.6 × 30) kJ

= 216 kJ

The total heat capacity of a 70 kg patient is 245 kJ °C^{-1}, as mentioned above, so the patient's mean temperature must fall by up to 1°C when 2 litres of unwarmed blood are transfused. Blood warmers are therefore advised when transfusions of this size are required.

Gases have low specific heats and this may be important in anaesthesia. Air, for instance, has a specific heat of 1.01 kJ kg^{-1} °C^{-1} at constant pressure. The quantity of a gas, however, is seldom measured in kilograms but usually expressed in terms of a volume. It is therefore more convenient to refer to the specific heat of a gas as the amount of heat required to raise the temperature of a unit volume of it by one temperature unit, i.e. the heat required to raise 1 litre of gas through 1 K (1°C). The low densities of gases mean that the specific heats expressed in this way are very low, e.g. the specific heat of air is only 1.2 J litre^{-1} °C^{-1}, about one-thousandth of the numerical value when expressed in terms of mass. The practical implication is that an extremely small quantity of heat is required or lost when the temperature of a small volume of a gas is altered. When a cigarette is smoked, for example, the burning tobacco is at a temperature of several hundred degrees Celsius. As air is drawn over this burning tobacco, it is heated to about this temperature. However, the temperature of this air falls dramatically by the time it reaches the mouth, even though the quantity of heat lost to the environment is small.

Another example, more appropriate to anaesthesia, concerns the temperature of the supply of anaesthetic gases to a patient. The gases at source may be quite cold if supplied directly from a vaporizer. As they pass through the anaesthetic breathing system, only a small quantity of heat is transferred, but this is sufficient to ensure that the gas is closer to ambient temperature by the time it arrives at the patient.

Normally the heat required to warm inspired air is quite small because of the low specific heat of the air. Consider a patient breathing at 7 litres min^{-1} with an endotracheal tube in the upper trachea. What is the heat loss from this source? The temperature in the upper trachea is about 34°C and so, if any heat exchange effect within the endotracheal tube is ignored, the temperature rise of the air could be 14°C, i.e. from a room temperature of 20°C to 34°C.

Heat loss from warming inspired air

$= $ Flow $\times$ Specific heat capacity $\times$ Temperature rise

$= 7$ litres $min^{-1} \times 1.2$ J litre^{-1} °C$^{-1} \times 14$°C

$= 118$ J min^{-1}

$= 1.96$ W $(1$ W $= 1$ J s$^{-1})$

As shown in the calculation, the heat loss is only about 2 W, an insignificant amount compared with the patient's heat loss in basal conditions of about 80 W. Consequently, heat loss from warming inspired air is not normally an important factor but, if dry gases are being inhaled, extra heat is needed to supply the latent heat to humidify the air.

Latent Heat

When a substance changes from a liquid to a vapour or from a solid to a liquid, heat must be supplied even though this change of state takes place at a constant temperature. The heat which is required is known as the latent heat of vaporization when the change is from a liquid to a vapour, or the latent heat of fusion when a solid changes to a liquid. Another category of latent heat is associated with a solid dissolving in or crystallizing out of a liquid, and is known as the latent heat of crystallization. Of these forms, the latent heat of vaporization is of most interest in anaesthesia.

Specific latent heat is defined as the heat required to convert 1 kilogram of a substance from one phase to another at a given temperature (SI unit of specific latent heat J kg^{-1}).

Figure 10.2 Specific latent heat of water at 100°C

Figure 10.3 Specific latent heat of water at 37°C

Thus, water at 100°C may be converted to steam at 100°C by supplying the appropriate quantity of latent heat, i.e. 2.26 MJ kg^{-1} water (Fig. 10.2). Note that the temperature at which the change of state occurs must be specified, because the value of latent heat depends on this.

At body temperature it is found that 2.42 MJ are required to turn 1 kg water into 1 kg vapour (Fig. 10.3). At room temperature the heat required is even greater: at 20°C, 2.43 MJ are needed, i.e. the lower the temperature the more latent heat is needed to vaporize a substance.

Figure 10.4 shows a graph of the change in latent heat with temperature for water. If this graph were extended to the right, the latent heat would continue to fall as the temperature rose, and would ultimately reach zero.

This is illustrated in the graph of the latent heat of vaporization of nitrous oxide (Fig. 10.5). The temperature at which the latent heat of vaporization of nitrous oxide becomes zero corresponds to its critical temperature of 36.5°C. At this temperature, the substance changes spontaneously from liquid to vapour without the supply of any external energy. Above this critical temperature the substance cannot exist as a liquid. Critical temperature is discussed in Chapter 4.

Latent Heat in Anaesthesia

A clinical example of latent heat of vaporization is seen in the use of ethyl chloride for local anaesthesia. Ethyl chloride is stored as a liquid under pressure in glass ampoules with a tap so that a fine jet of the substance may be directed onto the skin. Vaporization of the ethyl chloride causes pronounced cooling of the skin,

Figure 10.4 Specific latent heat of water as a function of temperature

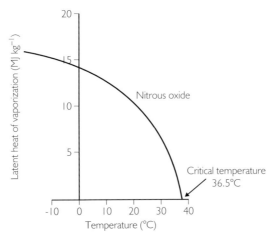

Figure 10.5 Specific latent heat of nitrous oxide as a function of temperature

thus impairing conduction in the sensory nerves and providing enough analgesia for minor surgical procedures such as the opening of a skin abscess or whitlow.

All volatile anaesthetic agents require latent heat for vaporization and this factor is important in the design of vaporizers. As gas passes over liquid anaesthetic in a vaporizer, the liquid vaporizes, taking latent heat of vaporization from the remaining fluid and from the surrounding vaporizer walls (Fig. 10.6). Thus, the temperature of the remaining anaesthetic agent and of the vaporizer walls falls. But a fall in temperature of the anaesthetic in the vaporizer renders it less volatile, lowering its saturated vapour pressure and so reducing the amount of anaesthetic vaporized.

Most vaporizers have systems for keeping the concentration of vapour constant. These systems are based on thermostatic devices, which are considered in Chapter 11.

Another effect of latent heat of vaporization can be seen if a nitrous oxide cylinder is allowed to empty rapidly (Fig. 10.7). Nitrous oxide is stored in cylinders in liquid form and, as it is used, it is converted to gas, the latent heat required being taken from the remaining fluid and from the cylinder walls. Thus, the temperature of the cylinder falls and water vapour from the air may condense or freeze on the outside of the cylinder. Because of the cooling, the vapour pressure falls rapidly inside such a cylinder and a pressure gauge, if fitted, gives a low reading which recovers towards the previous level after the cylinder is turned off, as shown by the dotted line in Fig. 10.7.

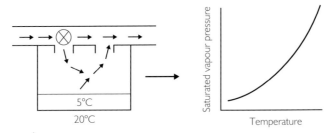

Figure 10.6 Effect of latent heat in a vaporizer

Figure 10.7 Change of pressure in a 900 litre nitrous oxide cylinder emptied at 5 litres min⁻¹; pressure is restored if the flow is turned off, as indicated by the dotted line

Carbon dioxide and cyclopropane are also stored in liquid form, but in normal anaesthetic practice the rate of use is so slow that cooling of the cylinder is not noticed.

Oxygen is another example of a gas which may be stored in liquid form in a hospital, as this is more economical. Because the critical temperature of oxygen is −119°C, it cannot exist as a liquid above this temperature.

In practice, the liquid oxygen in the storage vessel is at a temperature of around −160°C and must be kept in a special storage vessel resembling a gigantic vacuum flask to maintain it at this low temperature (Fig. 10.8). Normally the pressure inside the vessel is set to about 7 bar, this being the vapour pressure of the oxygen at −160°C.

When oxygen is taken from the top of the storage vessel, it is very cold and so it has to pass through a superheater coil, shown on the right of the diagram. Then it passes through a pressure regulator so that the pipeline pressure is kept at about 4.1 bar.

If oxygen flows at a fast rate, the temperature of the liquid oxygen falls because of the removal of latent heat and its vapour pressure falls. To solve this problem, a supplementary source of heat is needed and this is provided by a pressure raising vaporizer. A control valve senses the storage vessel pressure and controls the flow of liquid oxygen to the pressure-raising vaporizer – the lower the

Figure 10.8 Liquid oxygen supply system

pressure, the higher the flow of liquid oxygen. In the vaporizer, the oxygen is warmed and vaporized to the pipeline pressure.

No refrigeration unit is needed for the storage vessel because the liquid oxygen remains cold due to the efficiency of the vacuum container and the loss of latent heat as oxygen vaporizes. Nevertheless, if no oxygen is used the temperature of the storage vessel gradually rises until after about 1 week the oxygen pressure causes excess oxygen to be released through the safety valve. The evaporation of this liquid oxygen then reduces the temperature and pressure.

Latent Heat and Heat Loss from the Patient

The heat loss from warming inspired air has already been considered but not the heat loss for its humidification. By the time gases reach the trachea, their humidity is about 34 mg water vapour per litre of gas; this water comes from vaporization from the mucosa of the respiratory tract. Consider now a person breathing completely dry gases at 7 litres min^{-1}.

Humidity in the upper trachea $= 34$ mg $litre^{-1}$

Total water required to humidify inspired gas $= 7$ litres $min^{-1} \times 34$ mg $litre^{-1}$

$$= 0.238 \text{ g } min^{-1}$$

Total latent heat needed $=$ Specific latent heat of vaporization at $37°C \times$ Total water

$$= 2.42 \text{ MJ } kg^{-1} \times 0.000238 \text{ kg } min^{-1}$$

$$= 576 \text{ J } min^{-1}$$

$$= 9.6 \text{ W}$$

Specific heat to warm inspired air (calculated previously) $= 2.0$ W

Total heat loss from respiration $= 11.6$ W

As shown in the calculations, the heat lost in humidifying the air is much greater than that lost in warming dry air, and the total heat loss from respiration of almost 12 W represents 15% of the total basal heat loss of about 80 W.

This is a higher figure than the 10% given in Chapter 9 as a typical proportion of a person's heat production required for warming and humidifying typical room air during inspiration. In anaesthesia, however, the inspired gases are usually dry and consequently more heat is lost by this route than under normal conditions. This heat loss may contribute to the general problem of hypothermia during anaesthesia, especially in young children. It can be avoided by humidifying inspired gases and is reduced when an anaesthetic circle system with soda lime is used.

Vaporizers

11

A vaporizer is a device for adding clinically useful concentrations of anaesthetic vapour to a stream of carrier gas. Its use is necessary because the saturated vapour pressure of volatile anaesthetic agents at room temperature is many times greater than that required to produce anaesthesia. Since the introduction of vaporizers into anaesthetic practice, many different designs have been developed, not all of which are still in use. This chapter describes most of the current techniques and some of those that are no longer in use, the latter being included either because of their historical importance or the particular principle of their operation.

Plenum and Draw-Over Vaporizers

One of the most frequently used techniques is the mixing of carrier gas passing through a vaporizing chamber with gas containing no vapour to produce a final mixture with the appropriate concentration. This is achieved by splitting the flow of gas to the vaporizer into two streams, as shown in Fig. 11.1. One stream passes through the chamber containing the anaesthetic agent and the other bypasses it. These streams then reunite and pass to the patient.

Gas can be made to flow through a vaporizer in one of two ways. First, a positive pressure can be developed upstream of the vaporizer – e.g. by gas from a flowmeter – so that gas is pushed through. This type of vaporizer is known as a plenum vaporizer. Alternatively, as shown in Fig. 11.2, a subatmospheric pressure may be developed in the gas stream distal to the vaporizer, thus drawing gas through. This is known as a draw-over vaporizer and the subatmospheric pressure may be generated either by the patient's respiratory effort or by mechanical means. The plenum type of vaporizer is considered first.

From flowmeters

Figure 11.1 Principle of the plenum vaporizer

Figure 11.2 Principle of the draw-over vaporizer

The Boyle's Bottle

One of the earliest and simplest types of plenum vaporizer was the Boyle's bottle, illustrated in Fig. 11.3. The liquid anaesthetic agent is contained in a glass bottle and the proportion of gas flowing through the chamber relative to that flowing through the bypass is controlled by a rotary valve. In the illustration, the control lever for this valve is shown in the fully on position, and in this case all the gas flows directly over the surface of the anaesthetic agent. If the control lever is rotated downwards, part of the gas flow is diverted through the bypass channel shown and, in this way, the splitting ratio – i.e. the fraction of gas passing through the vaporizing chamber – may be varied.

In this vaporizer, the concentration of anaesthetic agent leaving the vaporizing chamber is very dependent on the flow; this concentration becomes less as the flow increases. To overcome this problem, the vaporizer is also fitted with a plunger and cowl which can direct the gas stream closer to the surface of the liquid or enable it to be bubbled through the liquid agent. The vaporizer thus has the inconvenience of requiring a second control to operate it, but this plunger is needed during induction to achieve an adequate concentration of an anaesthetic agent such as ether. If the Boyle's bottle is used for other anaesthetics for which high concentrations could be dangerous, the plunger is raised to its full extent.

This simple vaporizer has another problem, discussed in greater detail in Chapter 10. As the anaesthetic agent vaporizes, it draws latent heat of vaporization from the remaining liquid anaesthetic and from the walls of the vaporizer. The temperature and hence the saturated vapour pressure of the anaesthetic agent therefore fall. The concentration of anaesthetic from the vaporizer then decreases

Figure 11.3 The Boyle's bottle

unless readjustment of the settings is made. Because the output of the Boyle's bottle is so variable, it cannot be calibrated.

To a large extent, developments in vaporizer design have solved the problems of flow and temperature dependence and more accurate models have superseded the Boyle's bottle. These vaporizers are normally intended and calibrated for use with one anaesthetic agent only.

Flow Dependence

The problem of flow dependence may be overcome if it can be arranged that all the gas emerging from the vaporizing chamber is fully saturated at all flow rates. When this is the case, the final percentage of anaesthetic vapour delivered from the vaporizer can be controlled by adjustment of the splitting ratio and is independent of flow.

Figure 11.4 illustrates an isoflurane vaporizer at a room temperature of 20°C. The saturated vapour pressure of isoflurane at this temperature is 32 kPa. If the ambient atmospheric pressure is 100 kPa, i.e. 1 bar, the concentration of vapour in the vaporizing chamber is 32%, an example of Dalton's law of partial pressures. If the control valve is set to allow 5% of the incoming gas to flow through the chamber and 95% through the bypass channel, the resulting concentration of isoflurane is 1.6%. The concentration remains the same provided that the temperature is constant and the surface area of liquid isoflurane within the chamber is large enough to maintain the saturated vapour pressure.

The saturated vapour pressure of an anaesthetic agent such as isoflurane is greatly in excess of that required to maintain anaesthesia. If a fault occurs, e.g. in the control valve, an unintentionally high proportion of gas may pass through the vaporizing chamber and there is a risk of overdose and fatality. It is, therefore, essential for safety that the control valve and associated parts work reliably.

To achieve full saturation, a large surface area must be available for vaporization within the vaporizing chamber. One method of achieving this is to place metal or fabric wicks in the vaporizing chamber. One end of each of these wicks dips into the anaesthetic liquid, while the other end projects up into the chamber (Fig. 11.5A). Surface tension between the liquid anaesthetic and the capillary channels in the wicks draws the anaesthetic up, which provides a large surface area of anaesthetic and assists efficient vaporization.

An alternative method, shown in Fig. 11.5B, is to bubble the gas through the liquid anaesthetic agent by means of a sintered disc of glass or metal. This produces large numbers of minute bubbles which have a large total surface area. The copper kettle vaporizer employed this system.

Despite the use of a technique with full vapour saturation in the vaporizing chamber, circumstances can arise which affect a vaporizer's output. The splitting

Figure 11.4 Isoflurane vaporizer at 20°C and 100 kPa, illustrating principle of action

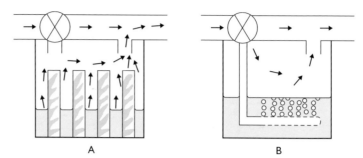

Figure 11.5 Techniques to achieve full saturation of gas in the vaporizing chamber:
(A) use of wicks and (B) use of small bubbles produced by sintered glass or metal

ratio produced in a particular vaporizer depends on the relative resistances to flow of the gas paths through the vaporizing chamber and through the bypass channel. These resistances depend on whether the flow is laminar, turbulent or a mixture of the two, and on the physical properties of the gases (e.g. viscosity and density). Flow dependence is usually worst at low flows, e.g. below 1 litre min^{-1}, and the manufacturer's calibration chart should be consulted if low flows are used. Care should be taken to ensure that the conditions under which the vaporizer is calibrated represent the clinical conditions under which it is used. A vaporizer which is calibrated with oxygen flowing through it will generally give a slightly different output with mixtures of nitrous oxide and oxygen.

The copper kettle series of vaporizers overcame these problems by using a flowmeter to control the flow of gas through the vaporizing chamber.

Temperature Stability

The glass of the Boyle's bottle and similar simple vaporizers is a poor conductor of heat and prevents effective conduction of heat from its surroundings. More advanced types of vaporizer are made of metal, which, having good thermal conductivity, allows heat to be transferred from the surroundings to the vaporizing chamber. In addition, the metal itself acts as a reservoir of heat to delay and reduce temperature fluctuations, as the heat capacity of the metal is added to that of the anaesthetic agent in the vaporizer (Fig. 11.6).

For example, consider a halothane vaporizer of 5 kg weight made of copper and containing 200 ml of halothane.

$$\text{Heat capacity of halothane} = \text{Volume} \times \text{Density} \times \text{Specific heat capacity}$$

$$= 200 \text{ ml} \times 1.87 \text{ g ml}^{-1} \times 0.8 \text{ J g}^{-1} \text{ K}^{-1}$$

$$= 299 \text{ J K}^{-1}$$

$$\text{Heat capacity of copper} = 5000 \text{ g} \times 0.39 \text{ J g}^{-1} \text{ K}^{-1}$$

$$= 1950 \text{ J K}^{-1}$$

$$\text{Total heat capacity} = 299 + 1950 \text{ J K}^{-1}$$

$$= 2249 \text{ J K}^{-1}$$

Although the specific heat of copper is not as high as that of halothane, copper is very dense and the large mass present in a typical vaporizer gives an important contribution to the heat capacity.

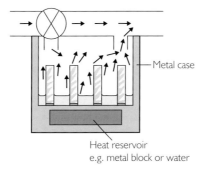

Figure 11.6 Partial control of temperature in a vaporizer by the use of a metal case and a heat reservoir

Water has an even higher specific heat capacity and it can also be used as a heat reservoir. The concept of a water reservoir is not new, as a container of water was sometimes used to surround a Boyle's bottle. If a Boyle's bottle contains 200 ml ether and the water reservoir is 200 ml, the calculations are as follows:

$$\text{Heat capacity of ether} = \text{Volume} \times \text{Density} \times \text{Specific heat capacity}$$

$$= 200 \text{ ml} \times 0.71 \text{ g ml}^{-1} \times 2.2 \text{ J g}^{-1} \text{ K}^{-1}$$

$$= 312 \text{ J K}^{-1}$$

$$\text{Heat capacity of water} = 200 \text{ ml} \times 1 \text{ g ml}^{-1} \times 4.18 \text{ J g}^{-1} \text{ K}^{-1}$$

$$= 836 \text{ J K}^{-1}$$

$$\text{Total heat capacity (excluding the glass vaporizer bottle)} = 312 + 836 \text{ J K}^{-1}$$

$$= 1148 \text{ J K}^{-1}$$

In practice, the thermal conductivity of glass is not as high as metal and this limits the temperature-stabilizing effect of the water bath.

Although the provision of heat reservoirs reduces the rate at which temperature changes occur, these changes are not eliminated.

Temperature Compensation

A graph of the relationship of temperature and saturated vapour pressure for isoflurane is illustrated in Fig. 11.7. At 20°C, the saturated vapour pressure is

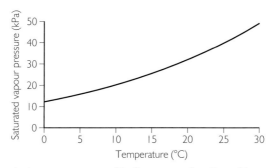

Figure 11.7 Saturated vapour pressure of isoflurane as a function of temperature

32 kPa, but at other temperatures this value is different. If the temperature of the anaesthetic agent in the vaporizing chamber falls, the concentration of anaesthetic vapour leaving the vaporizer also falls unless the splitting ratio of the gas is altered so that more gas flows through the vaporizing chamber. This adjustment, which is necessary to deliver a vaporizer output that does not depend on temperature, may be carried out manually or automatically.

In earlier models of the Dräger Vapor halothane vaporizer, the process was carried out manually. A thermometer was provided to monitor the temperature in the vaporizing chamber and a scale on the control knob allowed the anaesthetist to read the percentage of halothane accurately at a particular vaporizer temperature. This method allowed accurate concentrations of anaesthetic agent to be delivered.

The copper kettle vaporizer also had a system of manual adjustment, but here the two gas flows – through the bypass and through the vaporizing chamber – were entirely separate and were adjusted by separate flowmeters. The temperature in the vaporizer was noted and the flow rates through the vaporizer were adjusted according to a calibration chart to provide the required final concentration.

It is more convenient, however, for such an adjustment to take place automatically and most vaporizers contain a temperature-controlled valve which adjusts the splitting ratio. The control systems illustrated in Fig. 11.8 are shown acting on the flow through the vaporizers. However, in some vaporizers they operate instead on the bypass channel. One temperature-controlled valve incorporates a bimetallic strip, as shown in Fig. 11.8A. This consists of two metals which have different coefficients of thermal expansion and which are joined together. As the temperature changes, the shape of the strip alters, so that it bends or straightens. This strip may be used to operate a valve and is employed in several different vaporizers. Another method, illustrated in Fig. 11.8B, uses small flexible bellows containing fluid that has a high coefficient of expansion. As the temperature changes, the bellows expand or contract and thus open or close a valve. Alternatively, expansion and contraction of a metal rod can be used to adjust the valve (Fig. 11.8C).

The problems arising from the change of vapour pressure with temperature can be avoided if liquid anaesthetic is added directly to the gas stream. Several different techniques for doing this have been developed, one of which is shown in Fig. 11.9. The anaesthetic agent is delivered into the gas stream through a fine nozzle. The rate of delivery of the anaesthetic agent depends upon the pressure difference between P_1 and P_2 across the nozzle, and this is adjusted by the throttle valve. If flow through the vaporizer is increased, the pressure across the valve is increased and so more anaesthetic is delivered to maintain the same concentration. In this way the vaporizer remains accurate despite changes in flow, and the throttle valve is calibrated to indicate the percentage of anaesthetic delivered.

A   B   C

Figure 11.8 Temperature-controlled valves to adjust flow through the vaporizing chamber automatically based on (A) a bimetallic strip, (B) bellows and (C) a metal rod

Figure 11.9 Principle of injection of liquid anaesthetic agent

The heated-chamber pulsed vaporizer is shown in Fig 11.10. The anaesthetic agent bottle is pressurized, e.g. to 0.4 bar, which transfers the anaesthetic agent to a heated chamber. The temperature at the top of the chamber is accurately controlled by means of a heater and a thermistor temperature sensor.

Rearranging the ideal gas equation, $PV = nRT$, gives

$$\frac{n}{V} = \frac{P}{RT}$$

Thus the number of moles per unit volume is fixed if the pressure and temperature are constant.

A solenoid valve at the top of the vaporizing chamber alternately opens and closes. During the fixed opening period, a given volume, and therefore a given number of moles of anaesthetic agent, are added to the flow of fresh gas. The concentration of anaesthetic agent leaving the vaporizer is controlled by the frequency at which the valve is opened.

The vaporizer can only be used with a system that measures the fresh gas flow and produces an electronic output. This is then used to control the frequency at which the vaporizer valve is pulsed and hence maintain the desired vaporizer output concentration if the fresh gas flow is altered.

Desflurane Vaporizer

The anaesthetic agent desflurane has a boiling point of 22.6°C, so it requires a special design of vaporizer for its use. The principle of its operation is shown in Fig. 11.11.

Figure 11.10 Principle of the heated-chamber pulsed vaporizer

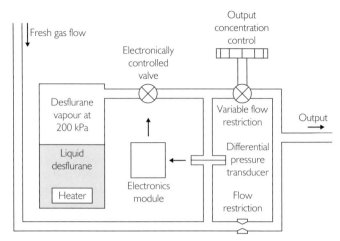

Figure 11.11 Principle of the desflurane vaporizer

The desflurane is held in a chamber heated to a temperature of 39°C, at which temperature the vapour pressure of desflurane is 200 kPa (2 bar). The fresh gas flow passes through a restriction on its way to the output of the vaporizer, which results in a rise in pressure upstream of the restriction. This pressure is measured by a differential pressure transducer and compared with the pressure resulting from the flow of desflurane through the variable restriction regulated by the output control knob set by the anaesthetist. The signal from the differential pressure transducer is processed electronically and used to adjust a valve upstream of the transducer in such a way that the differential pressure across the transducer remains at a predetermined value. Consequently, when the fresh gas flow is changed, the flow of desflurane changes to maintain the set concentration at the output where the two flows combine.

Effect of Pressure on a Vaporizer

The calibration of some vaporizers may be inaccurate during intermittent positive pressure ventilation (IPPV), and the vaporizer may give increased concentrations of anaesthetic, particularly if a low flow is used in association with IPPV with a closed circuit.

During IPPV, gas is supplied to the vaporizer at a constant rate which is set on the flowmeters on the anaesthetic machine, but intermittent back pressure from the ventilator can occur at the outlet of the vaporizer as the ventilator cycles. If the volume of the vaporizing chamber in the vaporizer is larger than the bypass channel, gas may expand out of the inlet and outlet of the vaporizing chamber when the back pressure from the ventilator falls. Thus, gas containing anaesthetic agent will flow into the bypass channel and increase the output concentration of the vaporizer.

This effect may be overcome in a number of ways. First, a pressurizing valve can be included downstream of the vaporizer to ensure that the pressure within the vaporizer is constant and greater than the pressure at the ventilator. Secondly, the vaporizer may be designed so that the volume of the bypass channel and vaporizing chamber are equal. If this is the case, expansion takes place equally from both routes and there is no retrograde flow. Thirdly, a long inlet tube to the vaporizing chamber can be provided so that retrograde flow from the vaporizing chamber never reaches the bypass channel.

A further problem has occurred in vaporizers subjected to pressure in that liquid anaesthetic has been decanted into the breathing system. This hazard is now avoided in the design of vaporizers.

Use at Hyperbaric Pressure

Anaesthetic vaporizers are also sometimes used at varying atmospheric pressure. Figure 11.12 illustrates the situation with a vaporizer set at 1% isoflurane. If the ambient atmospheric pressure is 100 kPa (1 bar), the partial pressure of isoflurane at the outlet is 1% of this, i.e. 1 kPa. At a room temperature of 20°C, the saturated vapour pressure of isoflurane in the vaporizer is 32 kPa, or 32% of the atmospheric pressure.

Consider what happens if this same vaporizer with the same setting is operated in a pressure chamber at 200 kPa (2 bar). The saturated vapour pressure is unaffected by ambient pressure; hence it is still 32 kPa, but this now constitutes 16% of the 200 kPa atmospheric pressure. Assuming that the splitting ratio is unchanged, there is, in addition to a halving of the percentage of isoflurane inside the vaporizer, a halving of the output percentage measured at the ambient 200 kPa pressure. The vaporizer is thus delivering 0.5% isoflurane at 200 kPa, which results in a partial pressure of isoflurane of 1 kPa, the same as before. As the depth of anaesthesia is dependent on the partial pressure of anaesthetic vapour rather than on its percentage, an anaesthetic vaporizer can normally be used with the usual settings at different atmospheric pressures.

Vaporizer Position and Controls

On the anaesthetic machine, a vaporizer should be placed between the flowmeter block and the emergency oxygen flush control (Fig. 11.13), so there is no risk that the high flow of oxygen from the latter can be delivered through the vaporizer. If there is a gas supply cut-out actuated by a failure of the oxygen supply, then this too is downstream from the vaporizer.

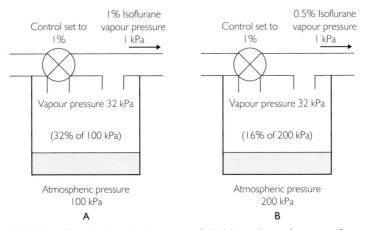

Figure 11.12 The effect of a hyperbaric pressure of 200 kPa on the performance of an isoflurane vaporizer; the percentage delivered is halved, but the partial pressure is unchanged

Figure 11.13 Aspects of vaporizer design and position

The vaporizer control knob should be standardized to turn to 'off' in a clockwise direction, as shown in Fig. 11.13. When the vaporizer is in the 'off' position, both the inlet and outlet ports to the vaporizing chamber should be occluded to avoid contamination of gas from the flowmeters with traces of anaesthetic.

Use of Vaporizers in Tandem

If two vaporizers are situated in tandem on the anaesthetic machine, the second one could become contaminated with vapour from the first. To solve this problem many manufacturers have an interlock mechanism which prevents two vaporizers being used simultaneously.

Draw-Over Vaporizers

The principles described for plenum vaporizers also apply to draw-over vaporizers, but the internal flow resistance of the draw-over vaporizer must be very low to avoid additional resistance to the patient's breathing. If such vaporizers are calibrated, they must retain their accuracy over a wide range of tidal ventilation. An example of the difficulty in achieving this arose in the special draw-over vaporizers which were used to give methoxyflurane or trichloroethylene as analgesics in obstetrics. In labour, patients tend to hyperventilate and early models of these vaporizers did not remain accurate during use.

At present, draw-over vaporizers are not generally used for analgesia, but some are used in portable anaesthetic apparatus. Because they do not require cylinder gas supplies, they are ideal for use outside hospital for emergencies, in major disasters or in remote areas.

The EMO (Epstein Macintosh Oxford) has a bellows thermal compensation device and is well established. It is heavier than the other vaporizers mentioned as it also has a water reservoir to aid thermal stability. It is designed for use with ether and, as this depresses the respiration less than isoflurane, it is safer for use in circumstances when oxygen is not available. The EMO, however, is less suitable for use with a continuous-flow plenum system as it then gives a lower percentage of anaesthetic than indicated.

The OMV (Oxford Miniature Vaporizer) is conveniently compact and has a small water reservoir but no thermal compensating valve. It is designed for use with halothane, trichloroethylene or enflurane, preferably with a system of oxygen supplementation. It can be used with a continuous or an intermittent flow, or with a draw-over technique. In a development of the OMV, the Triservice vaporizer, the heat-retaining reservoir contains antifreeze in place of water so that it is not damaged at low temperatures and continues to function in field use under winter conditions.

The PAC (portable anaesthesia complete) series of vaporizers have bimetallic strip temperature compensation, and their performance is not unduly affected by shaking, tilting or transient overturning – an advantage for vaporizers used in the field. Vaporizers are individually calibrated for the anaesthetic agent required and can be used in a plenum or draw-over system.

Draw-over vaporizers have also been used within an anaesthetic circle system using carbon dioxide absorption, but careful monitoring of the anaesthetic concentration is then needed as cumulative overdosage with the anaesthetic can occur, particularly if IPPV is used. In addition, contamination of the vaporizer with water vapour may affect its performance.

Care of Vaporizers

Most manufacturers recommend regular servicing of vaporizers, but the calibration of vaporizers can be checked with a refractometer (Chapter 13) or anaesthetic gas monitor if required. In the case of halothane and some other anaesthetics it is recommended that the vaporizer is drained and refilled at regular intervals, usually weekly, to prevent accumulation of preservatives such as thymol in the vaporizing chamber.

Care must be taken that calibrated vaporizers are filled only with the appropriate anaesthetic agent. To prevent accidental filling of vaporizers with the wrong liquid, a safety system is available using filler tubes and caps which only fit the appropriate vaporizers and bottles of anaesthetic agent.

Humidification

12

Humidification is of relevance to anaesthetists when considering patients whose normal humidifying mechanism in the nose and mouth has been bypassed, perhaps by tracheostomy or endotracheal intubation. As well as the benefit of humidification in protecting anaesthetized patients from drying of the mucosa of the trachea, humidification may reduce heat loss (Chapter 10) and may reduce the incidence of coughing and breath-holding during an inhalational induction.

In addition, humidity is of importance in the operating theatre because high humidity is unpleasant whereas low humidity may allow the accumulation of static charges with a risk of explosion if flammable agents are in use.

Units of Humidity

Humidity may be expressed in two ways. The first is the absolute humidity:

Absolute humidity is the mass of water vapour present in a given volume of air.

Values of absolute humidity are usually expressed as mg litre^{-1} or g m^{-3}, and these two measurements are numerically the same. The maximum amount of water vapour that can be present in a given volume of air is determined by the temperature.

As illustrated in Fig. 12.1, when temperature increases, the amount of water which can be present as vapour also increases. Hence fully saturated air at 20°C contains about 17 g m^{-3}, whereas at 37°C it contains 44 g m^{-3} when saturated.

The second way of measuring humidity, relative humidity, is a comparative method:

Relative humidity is the ratio of the mass of water vapour in a given volume of air to the mass required to saturate that given volume of air at the same temperature. It is usually expressed as a percentage.

From the graph (Fig. 12.1), it may be seen that 1 m^3 of air at 20°C, 100% saturated, contains about 17 g of water. If it is warmed to 37°C, the mass of water vapour or absolute humidity is still the same but the relative humidity is only 39%, as at 37°C, 1 m^3 of air contains 44 g of water vapour when fully saturated and the ratio of 17 to 44 gives a value of 39%.

Consider again the definition of relative humidity:

$$\text{Relative humidity} = \frac{\text{Mass present } M_P}{\text{Mass to saturate } M_S}$$

From the gas laws (Chapter 4):

$$n = \frac{PV}{RT}$$

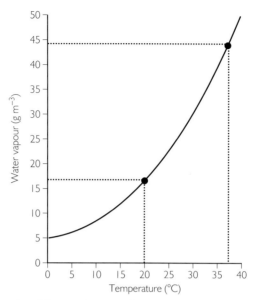

Figure 12.1 Absolute humidity as a function of temperature

and mass

$$M \propto n$$

where n is the number of moles, P is the absolute pressure, V is the volume, R is the universal gas constant, and T is the absolute temperature.

Therefore:

$$\text{Relative humidity} = \frac{\dfrac{P_p V}{RT}}{\dfrac{P_s V}{RT}}$$

If V, R and T are constant, then

$$\text{Relative humidity} = \frac{P_P}{P_S} = \frac{\text{Actual vapour pressure}}{\text{Saturated vapour pressure}}$$

It is seen that relative humidity can also be expressed as a ratio of vapour pressures.

Measurement of Humidity

Most instruments measure humidity as relative humidity. Figure 12.2 shows a hair hygrometer. It may be mounted on a wall of the operating theatre and gives a direct reading of relative humidity. The instrument uses the fact that a hair gets longer as the humidity rises, and the hair length controls a pointer moving over a scale. It has the advantage of simplicity, and is most accurate for relative humidities between 30 and 90%. Another form of meter works on a similar principle but has a special membrane in place of the hair.

Another instrument used for relative humidity measurement is the wet and dry bulb hygrometer (Fig. 12.3). It consists of two thermometers, as shown. The temperature of the mercury in the bulb on the right is in equilibrium with its

Figure 12.2 Hair hygrometer

surroundings and reads the true ambient temperature. However, the left thermometer reads a lower temperature because of the cooling effect from the evaporation of water from the wick surrounding its bulb and the consequent loss of latent heat of vaporization. The difference between the temperature registered by the two thermometers, ΔT, is related to the rate of evaporation of water which, in turn, depends on the ambient humidity. By using a set of tables it is possible to obtain relative humidity from this temperature difference. Notice that there must be sufficient air movement in the vicinity of the wet bulb to prevent a localized enhancement of humidity, and accurate instruments supply a controlled airflow over the thermometers.

A more accurate instrument for humidity measurement is Regnault's hygrometer (Fig. 12.4). It consists of a silver tube containing ether. To use the hygrometer, air is blown through the ether, cooling it and so initiating condensation on the shiny outside surface of the tube. The temperature at which condensation or misting occurs can then be noted and is known as the dew point, which is the temper-

Figure 12.3 Wet and dry bulb hygrometer

Figure 12.4 Regnault's hygrometer

ature at which the ambient air is fully saturated. Relative humidity may be deduced from the dew point as follows:

$$\text{Relative humidity} = \frac{\text{Actual vapour pressure}}{\text{SVP at that temperature}} = \frac{\text{SVP at dew point}}{\text{SVP at ambient temperature}}$$

where SVP is the saturated vapour pressure.

From a knowledge of the dew point and the saturated vapour pressures, which can be obtained from tables, both the relative and absolute humidities can be calculated at the temperature required.

Absolute humidity can also be measured by transducers, which are of two main types depending on the change either in electrical resistance or in capacitance of a substance when it absorbs water vapour from the atmosphere. The mass spectrometer (Chapter 20) has also been used in humidity studies and humidity can also be measured by a light absorption technique based upon the reduction of the ultraviolet light transmitted when water vapour is present.

Clinical Aspects of Humidity

When a patient breathes through the nose, the inspired air is warmed and saturated with water vapour before entering the trachea. If the nose is bypassed by an endotracheal tube or tracheostomy, dry air enters the trachea. The secretions present in the trachea may therefore become dried and tenacious and mucous plugs may form that block the respiratory tract. The secretions themselves are then more difficult for the patient to cough up or for the anaesthetist to aspirate. The cilia too may be inhibited or damaged by the dry gases, which also tend to have a chilling effect due to the latent heat lost from the mucosa as moisture evaporates to humidify the dry inspired gases. This inhibits ciliary activity further. If cilia are exposed to dry gases for a long period, they disappear and the epithelium of the trachea becomes keratinized. Such effects could occur in patients undergoing long-term intensive care but routine humidification has also been advocated for inhaled gases in anaesthesia. Normally, the air entering the upper trachea is saturated with water vapour to a humidity of 34 g m^{-3}, i.e. it is almost fully saturated at a temperature of 34°C. This provides a suitable level of humidity as a standard when humidifying inspired air in patients whose upper respiratory tract is bypassed, e.g. by a tracheostomy.

There are two methods of increasing the inspired humidity artificially. The first is by humidifying the environment, and the second is by humidifying the inspired gases

Figure 12.5 Heat and moisture exchanger (HME)

alone. Increases in total environmental humidity occur in infant incubators. In anaesthesia, however, humidifiers are commonly used to humidify the inspired gases alone.

Humidifiers

The simplest method of humidifying the inspired gases is the instillation of water droplets directly into the trachea, but this is the least satisfactory technique and cannot be recommended. It carries the danger that, if the drip is run too rapidly, the water or saline instilled into the trachea may lead to a condition similar to the acid-aspiration syndrome.

The heat and moisture exchanger (HME) provides another simple but more effective technique of humidification. Figure 12.5 shows one type of HME to illustrate its principle. It has an inlet and an outlet which form an enclosed unit. Inside this unit is a disposable element of paper, sponge, foam or fibre material impregnated with a hygroscopic substance such as calcium chloride, lithium chloride or silica gel. When the warm moist expired gas passes through this element, the gas is cooled and water condenses while the element is simultaneously warmed by the latent heat of the water condensing on it and by the exhaled gas. During inspiration the reverse process occurs: the moisture evaporates, humidifying the inspired gas and, since the element has been warmed above room temperature, the inspired gas is also warmed.

As this technique of conservation of moisture occurs in the nose, this humidifier has been called the 'artificial nose'. The name 'condenser humidifier' has also been used. The efficiency of the humidifier will depend on the ambient temperature; thus, in a hot climate there may be little temperature change within the hygroscopic element and negligible condensation. Under optimum conditions, however, an inspired air humidity of over $25\ g\ m^{-3}$ may be achieved with some types of HME.

At high minute volumes, the HME is less efficient and a general problem with HMEs is that secretions may be deposited on the moisture exchanging element, particularly if the patient coughs, increasing the resistance to breathing and the risk of infection with organisms such as pseudomonas. Frequent changes of the humidifier are therefore recommended by manufacturers.

A variant of the HME is available which includes a bacterial filter; it is known as the heat and moisture exchanging filter (HMEF) and is used to isolate infected patients from breathing systems and to protect patients who are particularly vulnerable to infection.

Another system of humidification uses a water bath; in its simplest form this system consists of dry gases bubbling through water at room temperature, but there are then two main disadvantages. First, such a system lacks efficiency

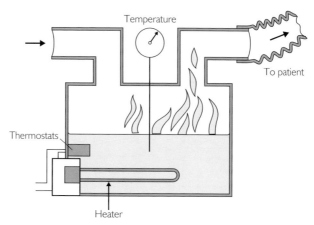

Figure 12.6 Hot water bath humidifier

because of the large bubbles, although by passing the gas through sintered glass to reduce the bubble size, the efficiency can be increased. The second problem is the loss of heat from the water by latent heat of vaporization, resulting in cooling, which reduces the humidity obtainable. This problem of cooling is overcome by adding an electric heater, which can also obviate the need to bubble the gas stream through the water (Fig. 12.6), and adjustment of the water bath temperature gives flexibility in the amount of water vapour which can be added to the gas stream.

The temperature at which the humidifier is operated depends on the humidity required at the patient and the temperature drop along the tubing. The operating temperature is normally about 40–45°C, but higher temperatures up to 60°C may sometimes be employed to prevent the growth of bacteria within the humidifier. There is a danger of scalding the patient if too high a temperature is present. This risk may be further increased in the case of patients receiving intermittent positive pressure ventilation (IPPV), especially if a ventilator fault occurs that results in a sudden increase in flow through the humidifier.

If the patient continuously inspires fully saturated gas at body temperature or higher, the heat normally lost via the respiratory tract in the warming and humidification of the inspired air is prevented. Heat may even be added to the patient and, if other physiological methods of heat loss are depressed and inadequate, hyperthermia may occur, especially in young children.

To avoid the dangers of overheating of the humidifier, a thermostat is present (Fig. 12.6). If the water overheats, the thermostat automatically switches off power to the heater. There is usually also a second thermostat in reserve in case the first fails, as well as a thermometer to indicate the temperature of the humidifier.

A potential problem with this humidifier is illustrated in Fig. 12.7. The water vaporized can condense in a redundant loop of the delivery tubing and obstruct the gas flow to the patient; such a pool of hot water could even be blown into a patient's tracheostomy. It is important, therefore, to ensure that the water condensing out can run back to the humidifier or into a water trap.

Figure 12.8 illustrates further refinements to the heated water bath principle. This is the cascade humidifier, in which gas bubbles through a perforated screen at the bottom of a wide tube, causing a foam of water and gas to pass up the tube. The large surface area of gas exposed to the water ensures that the gas is fully humidified. The thermistor positioned at the patient connection on the right of the

Figure 12.7 Condensation of water in a loop of delivery tube from a hot water bath humidifier

Figure 12.8 Cascade humidifier

figure monitors the temperature of the gases delivered and controls the heater element in the water bath to maintain an optimum delivery temperature and avoid any risk of burns to the patient. This gives safer and more accurate control than is possible when the water bath temperature alone is monitored. As the gases are fully saturated, the temperature at the patient also indicates absolute humidity at this point.

An alternative technique for adding water as vapour is the heated element humidifier illustrated in Fig. 12.9. Water is vaporized by dripping it on to an electric element heated to 100°C, the high temperature ensuring sterility. Also shown is a water trap which collects excess water. In an alternative form of this device, small pulsed volumes of water are delivered to the heated element and an element temperature of 250°C is used. However, humidifiers with such hot elements are less suited to use with anaesthetic vapours or volatile drugs as the heat may cause chemical changes. The amount of water vapour delivered from these humidifiers must be controlled according to the minute volume and humidity required, and a thermistor at the patient connector may be present to assist this control and avoid any risk of burns.

Figure 12.9 Heated element humidifier

Nebulizers

The nebulizer is another form of humidifier and may be of two types: gas-driven or ultrasonic.

The gas-driven nebulizer depends on the Bernoulli effect and the process of jet entrainment (Chapter 2). A high-speed flow of gas causes a drop in pressure at the end of a tube, which allows water to be drawn up and entrained from the tube (Fig. 12.10). The entrained water is then broken up into a spray of droplets of various sizes by the fast-moving gas stream. If the gas stream hits an anvil, as shown, the larger droplets can be baffled out or divided into smaller droplets.

Because some of the water from the droplets vaporizes and absorbs latent heat, there is a fall of temperature in the humidifier, so its effectiveness can be increased by adding a heater. A further problem with this type of nebulizer is that back pressure may alter the entrainment ratio, and can therefore affect the efficiency of the device.

Figure 12.10 Gas-driven nebulizer

To patient

Plate vibrating at ultrasonic frequency
(e.g. 2MHz)

Figure 12.11 Ultrasonic nebulizer

In the ultrasonic form of nebulizer, the droplets of water are formed by a vibrating surface (Fig. 12.11). The water may be dropped on a vibrating surface or formed from a pool lying on such a surface. The frequency of vibration is usually a few megahertz, which produces extremely small droplets.

The size of the droplets produced by a nebulizer is important. It has been shown that droplets of over 20 microns (μm), if not baffled out, are a nuisance as they fall out to form pools of water either in the tubing or in the upper respiratory tract. Droplets of 5 μm fall out in the region of the trachea, whereas any particles of 1 μm tend to pass right through to the alveoli and be deposited there. Droplets below 1 μm in size tend to be extremely stable and can be inspired and then expired again. One micron is ideal and ultrasonic nebulizers are most efficient at producing this size of water droplet, but slightly larger particle sizes may be helpful to loosen secretions in the trachea.

By the addition of droplets to the inspired gas, it is relatively easy to obtain moisture levels corresponding to relative humidities of well over 100%, and so, especially with children, it is easy to overload the patient with water, which may cause pulmonary oedema. The inspired droplets also increase the density of the gases and raise the resistance to turbulent flow.

One further point to note is that, as small droplets are stable and can carry for long distances, they may be a prolific source of cross-infection, particularly if a humidifier becomes infected. Solutions used in the humidifier must be sterile and the humidifier kept free from contamination.

Relative Efficiency of Humidifiers

A diagram of the approximate efficiencies of the various humidifiers is illustrated in Fig. 12.12, in which absolute humidity readings are used to avoid the need to specify the temperature. There are vertical dotted lines at 34 g m^{-3}, representing the normal level of humidity in the upper trachea, and at 44 g m^{-3}, representing full saturation at 37°C.

Figure 12.12 Approximate efficiency of humidifiers; the exact values depend on the model of humidifier in use

The unheated humidifier is not very efficient. The heat and moisture exchanger is more efficient, but it must be changed frequently.

The heated water bath humidifier and the heated Bernoulli type of nebulizer provide humidity close to that normally present in the upper trachea. The ultrasonic nebulizer is the most efficient method of adding water to the inspired gases, but it is expensive. Its efficiency also leads to the need for special care to avoid overdosage.

Finally, the problem of cross-infection must always be remembered, regardless of the type of humidifier used.

The Sine Wave and Wave Patterns

13

The Concept of a Sine Wave

In medicine, there are various biological processes that occur in a repetitive manner, e.g. the ventilation of the lungs and the cardiac cycle. When these are monitored, a complex wave pattern is seen. Figure 13.1 shows tracings of arterial pressure, of the electrocardiogram (ECG), and of the electroencephalogram (EEG), and gives examples of different types of simple waveforms: the sine wave, the sawtooth wave and the square wave. Of these, the sine wave is of special importance because it is possible to produce any of the other patterns by combining together various different sine waves.

Wave motion is also present as variation in pressure in the case of sound waves and variation in the electric and magnetic fields in the case of electromagnetic radiation such as light.

Two illustrations of sine wave production are given in Fig. 13.2. On the right, the movement of the coil in an electrical generator produces a sine wave pattern of electric current. This type is known as alternating current (AC) electricity, and is discussed in Chapter 14. Sine waves may also be produced mechanically and, in both cases, the principle involved is the same. Illustrated on the left of Fig. 13.2 is a pump with a piston moving up and down with the movement of a crankshaft. At the bottom of the diagram, the rotation of the crankshaft produces a vertical displacement, d, and if the vertical movement of this crankshaft is traced against time a sine wave is produced.

As shown in Fig. 13.3, the vertical displacement d and the angle of the crankshaft A form a right-angled triangle with the crankshaft of fixed length r as the

Figure 13.1 Wave patterns

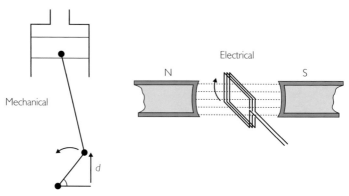

Figure 13.2 Sine wave production

hypotenuse. The sine of the angle A is equal to d/r so, regardless of the position of the crank at any time, the distance d is equivalent to $r \sin A$. Angle A has a different value at each moment because the crank is rotating at a constant rate and so a graph can be obtained with the displacement d on the vertical axis and the angles of A corresponding to the different times along the horizontal axis. This results in a sine wave pattern, as shown on the right of Fig. 13.3.

Characteristics of a Sine Wave

Phase

The different angles of A along the horizontal axis are referred to as the phase of the sine wave. One complete rotation of the pump crankshaft results in one complete cycle on the graph, and so 360° corresponds to one complete cycle (Fig. 13.4). A rotation of the crank through 180° is half a cycle and through 90° a quarter of a cycle.

If two sine wave motions are compared, as shown on the graph (Fig. 13.5), the relative displacement of one wave with respect to the other can be referred to

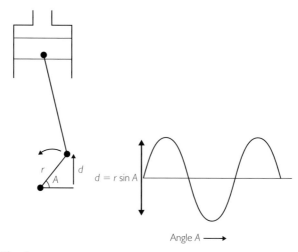

Figure 13.3 The sine wave

Figure 13.4 Phase of a sine wave

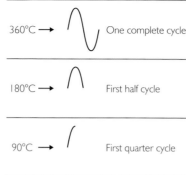

360°C → One complete cycle

180°C → First half cycle

90°C → First quarter cycle

in terms of the number of degrees by which the two waves differ along the horizontal axis. In the example illustrated, the two sine waves differ by exactly one-quarter of a cycle or 90°, so they are said to be 90° out of phase.

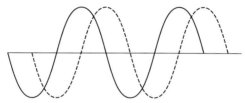

Figure 13.5 The two sine waves illustrated are 90° out of phase

Wavelength and Amplitude

Consider now the sine wave shown in Fig. 13.6. The wavelength is the distance between any two corresponding points in successive cycles, i.e. the distance between two peaks or two troughs, or the distance between two points where the wave motion cuts the horizontal axis in the same direction. The maximum displacement of the wave from the horizontal axis is known as its amplitude, and is also marked on the illustration. In the case of sound waves, a large amplitude is loud and a small amplitude quiet, whereas with light waves a large amplitude is bright and a small amplitude dim.

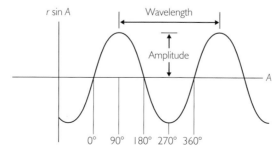

$r \sin A$ Wavelength

Amplitude

A

0° 90° 180° 270° 360°

Figure 13.6 Wavelength and amplitude

Frequency, Period and Velocity

The frequency of a wave is the name given to the number of complete cycles which occur in 1 second, and in the SI system the unit of measurement for cycles per second is given the name hertz and is denoted by the symbol Hz.

In Fig. 13.7, the waveform has a frequency of 10 cycles per second or 10 hertz and, as 10 complete cycles occur in 1 second, the time taken for each cycle is one-tenth of a second. The time taken for one complete cycle to occur is referred to as the period of the wave motion and is the reciprocal of the frequency:

$$T = \frac{1}{f}$$

where T is the period and f is the frequency.

Consider now the velocity of a wave motion:

Velocity = Frequency × Wavelength

Figure 13.7 illustrates a wave motion with a frequency of 10 Hz. If it has a wavelength of 1 m, the velocity of the wave motion is then 10 m s^{-1}.

Different wave motions have different velocities; sound, for example, has a velocity of 330 m s^{-1} in air. If the velocity is fixed, then frequency and wavelength are interrelated: the higher the frequency, the shorter the wavelength and vice versa.

Sound waves of different frequencies are heard as different pitches; for example, a sound wave with a high frequency has a short wavelength and a high-pitched note, whereas a sound with a low frequency has a longer wavelength and sounds low pitched. The behaviour of light can also be explained in terms of wave motion. A light wave with a high frequency and a short wavelength is seen as blue, whereas one with a lower frequency and longer wavelength appears red.

Visible light is a small part of the electromagnetic spectrum, which also includes radio waves, infrared and ultraviolet radiation, X-rays and gamma rays, as illustrated in Fig. 13.8. The velocity of electromagnetic radiation is constant in a vacuum for all frequencies and is equal to 3×10^8 m s^{-1}. In solids and liquids, it is slower, but in gases such as air the reduction in velocity is so small that the wavelength can be regarded as the velocity in a vacuum divided by the frequency, as shown in the figure. It is usual to describe electromagnetic waves in particular parts of the spectrum in different ways. Radio waves are quoted as a frequency, up to 10^9 Hz (1 GHz), and infrared, visible and ultraviolet radiations as a wavelength, usually in μm or nm. For X-rays and gamma rays a unit of energy called the electronvolt (eV) is used (see Appendix), the energy of a wave being equal to a constant times its frequency. X-rays and gamma rays of clinical interest have energies ranging from keV to MeV.

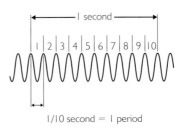

Figure 10 Hz = 10 cycles per second

Figure 13.7 Period and frequency

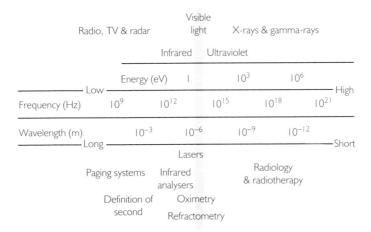

Figure 13.8 Electromagnetic spectrum

Various uses of the different electromagnetic radiations are made in medicine. Both staff paging systems and the technique of remote monitoring by telemetry use radio waves. Gases are capable of absorbing electromagnetic radiation and use has been made of this fact to produce infrared meters for carbon dioxide and nitrous oxide analysis. Infrared radiation is also used to form images in thermography. Gamma rays and X-rays are essential to radiology and are used in radiotherapy and nuclear medicine. Visible light is also used in many medical instruments, e.g. in the oximeter used to measure oxygen saturation in blood (Chapter 18) and in refractometry, considered later. Lasers (Chapter 24) use light in the visible and infrared wavelengths.

Gases emit electromagnetic radiation if they are suitably excited, e.g. by bombardment by electrons, and the wavelengths of radiation emitted are characteristic of the gas. In the SI system, the second is defined in terms of the frequency of radiation emitted by atoms of caesium-133.

The Doppler Effect

An example of the Doppler effect is the change in the pitch of sound emitted from a rapidly moving vehicle as it passes the observer. As mentioned above, if the pitch of a note changes, a change in frequency must have occurred. Consider now how this happens. Sound waves are regions of high and low pressure in the air, and they travel through it at a fixed velocity. At the top of Fig. 13.9 is a stationary source of sound emitting sound waves of a particular frequency. The separation between high- and low-pressure regions depends on the wavelength and therefore on the frequency. Now suppose the source, still emitting the same frequency, starts moving towards the listener. In the interval between producing high-pressure regions, the source has moved forward and so each high-pressure region becomes closer to the previous one. Consequently, the wavelength of this sound becomes shorter. Because of the relationship between wavelength and frequency, the ear of the listener picks up this shorter wavelength as an increase in frequency compared with the same source when stationary and the pitch of the note is higher. Conversely, as a source moves away from a listener, it is heard as a lower pitch because of the decrease in frequency. These changes in frequency constitute the Doppler effect.

Figure 13.9 Doppler effect

Various uses are made of the Doppler effect in medicine. One application is the ultrasonic blood flow detector (Fig. 13.10). Ultrasound is very high frequency sound which is above the range of human hearing but which travels well through body tissues. In this apparatus, ultrasonic waves from a vibrating crystal trans-mitter are beamed along an artery and the red blood cells reflect these high-frequency sound waves. A receiving transducer, incorporated into the pencil-like head of the apparatus, detects the reflected sound waves and, because of the movement of the red blood cells, these reflected sound waves have a Doppler change in frequency. This change in frequency is sensed electronically and is related to the velocity of the blood cells. Although it is difficult to calibrate the apparatus to provide quantitative measurements of blood flow, this technique can detect blood flow in an artery and is used to provide a qualitative assessment of the degree of success of arterial grafts, especially in the leg. The human ear can-not detect this high-frequency ultrasound but the apparatus often incorporates a system to produce audible sound related to the flow velocity. If the detector is used with a recorder, analysis of the tracing gives additional information regard-ing the flow pattern through the artery.

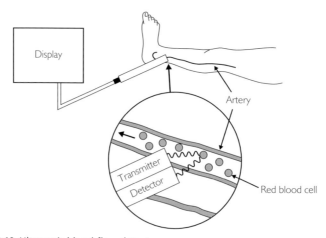

Figure 13.10 Ultrasonic blood flow detector

A similar type of apparatus using the same principle has been designed to assess blood flow in other vessels; for example, an indication of cardiac output may be obtained if a detector is used to monitor the velocity of the blood in the arch of the aorta. In order to make this measurement, the diameter of the aorta has to be known, since, for the same velocity, the volume flow measured in litres per minute is lower in a narrow vessel than in a wide vessel.

A similar type of apparatus is used in obstetrics to monitor the fetal heart rate during labour (Fig. 13.11). In this case the equipment detects the ultrasound beam after it has been reflected off the moving fetal heart. The apparatus consists of transmitting and receiving transducers which are placed on the abdominal wall and which may comprise separate units as shown or a single piezoelectric crystal used for both functions. The equipment permits any change in the fetal heart rate during labour to be detected more rapidly and more accurately than by the usual method of auscultation. In addition, the apparatus may be used to detect and measure the fetal heart rate in early pregnancy.

When sound waves, or other types of wave, reach a boundary between two different substances, part of the wave is transmitted and part reflected. In the case of sound waves, it is the difference in density between the two materials which determines the proportions of the wave which are transmitted and reflected. If an ultrasound transducer is used to transmit and receive sound waves into and out of the body, the waves must pass several times between air, which has a low density, and solid structures, which have a high density. This results in severe attenuation of the signal. Smearing gel on the surface of the skin and placing the transmitting face of the transducer in this gel reduces the difference in densities of the materials through which the ultrasound travels and greatly reduces the attenuation of the wave, thereby improving the performance of the ultrasound equipment.

Ultrasound waves are also used to form images of body structures because the waves are reflected off boundaries and interfaces between substances of different densities. In this case, the same transducer is used to transmit and receive the ultrasound waves and it is not the Doppler effect but the time taken for the ultrasound wave to travel from the transducer and return which allows the depth of a boundary or change in density to be measured. The transducer can be moved to and fro through an arc by a small motor so that the ultrasound beam scans a sector of the body and enables a cross section of the body to be displayed. Alternatively, a transducer comprised of many small individual crystals arranged in a line may be used to display a cross section through the body. Ultrasound imaging equipment is used

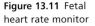
Figure 13.11 Fetal heart rate monitor

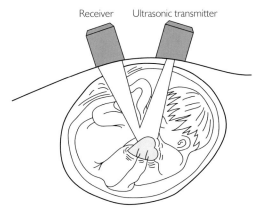

Receiver   Ultrasonic transmitter

for general abdominal examination and in specialities such as obstetrics and gynaecology, cardiology (where the scan is known as an echocardiogram) and urology.

Some ultrasound imaging equipment also provides a coloured map of blood flow, obtained by means of the Doppler effect and overlaid on the image of the body structures.

When the body is exposed to ultrasound, some of the sound energy is absorbed by the tissues. Ultrasound therapy units generate ultrasound of high intensity and are used to provide local heating as a physiotherapy treatment. In all applications of ultrasound, there is a limit to the power which can be absorbed by the tissues without adverse effect, as the absorbed power produces a rise in temperature. If very high power is used, the pressure in the sound wave can fall to zero during the minimum of the waveform and this can result in the rapid creation and collapse of bubbles in the tissues, a potentially damaging process known as cavitation.

Interference

Consider what happens when two or more sine waves are added together. Figure 13.12 shows on the left the result of adding two sine waves which have the same frequency, amplitude and phase. The resultant sine wave has a greatly enhanced amplitude. On the other hand, if these two sine waves are 180° out of phase, the resultant sine wave has zero amplitude and appears as a straight line, as shown on the right of the figure.

This interaction of two such sine waves is called interference and the resultant wave depends on the phase of the two wave motions which interfere. This phenomenon is used in optical devices for analysing various gases or vapours. An example is the refractometer, sometimes called the interferometer, with which the concentration of halothane in oxygen may be measured and the performance of vaporizers checked. Two light beams pass through the refractometer, one through a sample chamber and one through a reference chamber (Fig. 13.13).

Consider what happens when these two beams are now added together. Either they arrive at a point with their wave motions in phase, in which case reinforcement takes place and the increased amplitude gives rise to a bright fringe, or they combine out of phase and the reduced amplitude gives rise to a dark fringe. Thus, as shown on the right of Fig. 13.13, an array of light and dark fringes results. Suppose the reference chamber is left unchanged and an unknown concentration of sample gas added to the sample chamber. This reduces the velocity of the light passing through the sample chamber and alters the phase relationships when the two light beams are recombined, and so a displacement of the fringe pattern occurs which can be observed through an eye piece. The displacement of a selected fringe is directly proportional to the concentration of gas added to the sample chamber.

Figure 13.12 Addition of sine waves of same frequency and amplitude

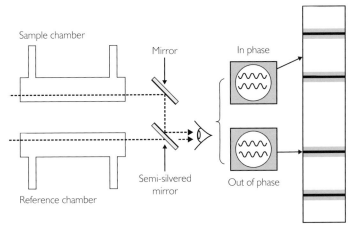

Figure 13.13 Principle of the refractometer

Small portable refractometers may be used to measure gas concentrations, but more sensitive versions also exist. The refractometer is nonspecific and may be used for measuring the concentration of a variety of different gases. On the other hand, it cannot be used to identify component gases in a mixture and so these must be known in advance.

For example, when a refractometer is used to check the performance of a vaporizer, the refractometer calibration using a mixture of halothane and oxygen is not identical with that for a mixture of halothane in nitrous oxide and oxygen.

Interference Filters

The phenomenon of interference is used in the interference filter, an optical component used to select one wavelength from a spectrum of wavelengths.

Electromagnetic radiation is partially reflected when it strikes a boundary between two media. The fractions transmitted and reflected depend on the characteristics of the media, the wavelength of the radiation and the angle of incidence. An interference filter is a block of material which is transparent to the radiation of interest and which has been coated with a very thin layer of a different transparent material. A proportion of the radiation passing through this coating is reflected at both surfaces of the coating and rejoins radiation which has passed straight through. The radiation which has been reflected twice interferes with the radiation which has passed straight through, the two beams being in phase only if the wavelength is a multiple of twice the thickness of the coating. Therefore only radiation with a multiple of twice the coating thickness will pass through with little attenuation. For other wavelengths the two beams will be out of phase and the intensity of the transmitted radiation will be reduced. Radiation which passes through a thin transparent coating of this type is therefore filtered and the arrangement is known as an interference filter. Filters of this type are useful for selecting the required wavelength of infrared radiation for use in an infrared analyser (Chapter 19).

The Frequency Spectrum

Figure 13.14 illustrates the results of adding sine waves with differing frequencies and amplitudes, as well as a differing phase relationship. It is seen that the resultant

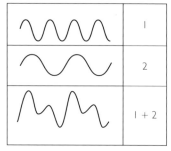

Figure 13.14 Addition of sine waves of differing frequencies and amplitudes

waveform is no longer a sine wave but in this case is a wave pattern similar to an arterial pressure tracing. This result is obtained simply by adding the amplitudes of the component waves at every point along their cycles.

The addition of whole ranges of sine waves, each with a different frequency, amplitude and phase, may result in quite complex waveforms and, as an example, Fig. 13.15 shows how an ECG waveform could be produced by adding a large range of frequencies. The range of these frequencies is important in the design and use of monitoring apparatus and may be described by a spectrum of frequencies.

In such a spectrum (Fig. 13.16) the ECG is composed of a range of frequencies from about 0.5 to 100 Hz, whereas an EEG signal has a smaller range of frequencies. The slower waves of the EEG are only about 1–5 Hz, whereas the faster beta waves are in the range of 15–60 Hz. In the EMG (electromyogram), there are sharp spikes and these indicate high-frequency components as shown.

Figure 13.15 Component frequencies of the ECG

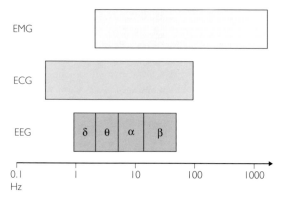

Figure 13.16 Frequency distribution of three biological electrical signals

Any waveform, no matter how complex, can be produced by selecting and adding together appropriate sine waves. The mathematical process of analysing complex wave patterns into a series of simpler sine wave patterns is called Fourier analysis, and this concept helps in understanding the patterns of biological electrical signals. The two main points to note are that, firstly, any complex wave pattern may be analysed into a large number of sine wave components and, secondly, wave patterns that have sharp spikes in them have high-frequency components, whereas smooth and rounded wave patterns consist of a more limited range of frequencies.

Electricity

14

Static Electricity and Electrical Potential

The word electricity is derived from 'elektron', the Greek word for amber. As with all substances, the atoms in amber consist of a positively charged nucleus surrounded by negatively charged electrons. Rubbing amber against another material can lead to a transfer of electrons, so that one of the substances will have an excess of them and the other a deficit. This phenomenon may also occur with other substances – e.g. plastics and rubber – and is known as static electricity. Such static electricity can be a source of ignition in anaesthetic explosions (Chapter 23). Static electricity is not the only cause of one object having an excess of electrons and another a deficit: this phenomenon also occurs as a result of chemical reactions in batteries, and in biological tissues. The electrons in the objects with the excess then possess potential energy in the same manner that the height of an object determines its gravitational potential energy. There is said to be an electric potential difference between the object with the excess and that with the deficit.

Conductors, Insulators and Semiconductors

Under the influence of a potential difference (or a changing magnetic field, dealt with below) electrons can pass from one atom to another and an electric current is the movement of such electrons through a substance. Substances may be classified into conductors, insulators or semiconductors, according to their ability to conduct electrons.

Conductors are usually metals, although certain other substances such as carbon are also good conductors. The outer electrons of atoms of a metal are loosely bound and can readily move through the metal under the influence of an electric potential. Some liquids, such as saline and body fluids, can also conduct electricity, as they contain positive and negative charged ions, which can move easily in response to an electric potential.

In insulators the electrons are firmly bound and therefore not normally able to move and form an electric current.

Semiconductors are used in components such as thermistors, transistors and diodes. The conductivity of semiconductors is intermediate between that of conductors and insulators. In a semiconductor, the outer electrons are bound to atoms less firmly than in an insulator. This means that by giving such an electron a little extra energy it can escape from the atom it is bound to and hence conduct electricity. This phenomenon is used in many devices. In a thermistor, heat is the source of energy. As the temperature increases, more electrons escape and hence the conductivity increases. The thermistor can be calibrated to measure temperature (Chapter 9). On the other hand excessive heat will adversely affect the performance of anaesthetic monitoring equipment containing semiconductors.

A photodetector is a special type of semiconductor in the form of a resistor, diode or transistor. When radiation falls on the detector, electrons in the material absorb some of the energy of radiation and are able to move through the material more freely. The photodetector is connected in an electronic circuit in which the electrons that have absorbed the light energy cause a change in current as light falls on the device.

Magnetic Field

A conductor with a current flowing through it can exert a force on another conductor carrying a current; this is the property known as magnetism. Some substances, e.g. iron alloys, can exhibit magnetism although it appears that no current is flowing through them. In this case, the magnetism is due to the sum of the many minute currents formed by the motion of electrons orbiting their nuclei.

The region throughout which a magnet or a current-carrying conductor exerts its effects is known as a magnetic field, and a changing magnetic field induces a flow of electrons in a conductor to produce an electric current.

If a conductor is wound into a coil, a current flowing in it produces a magnetic field which is strongest within the core of the coil. The strength of this magnetic field can be increased if a piece of a suitable magnetic material such as iron is placed into the core of the coil. Substances which possess this property are known as ferromagnetic materials; a further property of ferromagnetic materials is that they are strongly attracted into a magnetic field.

The term magnetic field strength is used to describe the power of the field in a vacuum; the term magnetic flux describes the field which results when a magnetic field is present in any material and, as noted above, this may be greater than the original magnetic field strength. In general, magnetic flux is increased greatly over magnetic field strength in ferromagnetic materials, increased slightly in paramagnetic materials and decreased in diamagnetic materials.

The unit of magnetic flux is the weber (Wb), being that flux which, when linked with a single turn, generates an electromotive force (emf) of 1 volt in the turn, as it decreases uniformly to zero in 1 second. The unit of magnetic flux density is the tesla (T), being $Wb\ m^{-2}$. The magnetic flux density produced in air by the earth's magnetic field is approximately 60 μT, whereas the powerful magnetic fields used by magnetic resonance imaging (MRI) equipment are generally in the range 0.2–4 T.

Direct and Alternating Current

The term direct current (DC) describes a steady flow of electrons along a wire or through a component in one direction only (Fig. 14.1). Sources of direct current include thermocouples (Chapter 9) and batteries.

In a battery, chemical energy is converted into electrical energy through a chemical reaction. In a non-rechargeable battery or primary cell, the chemical reaction is not reversible but in a rechargeable battery or secondary cell, the chemical reaction is reversible by the passage of current in a direction opposite to that in which it is supplied by the battery. Rechargeable batteries are used in many items of portable equipment in order that the equipment can be used when a mains supply is not readily available. A battery charger is usually included in or with the equipment so that the batteries may be recharged from the mains supply and are always ready for use. Primary cells should never be used to replace rechargeable batteries unless equipment is specifically designed to allow this. An attempt to recharge a primary cell will result in the generation of gas and the destruction of the cell; an explosion may also occur.

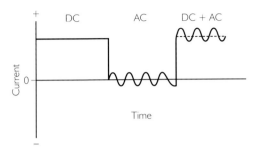

Figure 14.1 Current as a function of time for direct current, alternating current and a combination of the two

The term alternating current (AC) describes a flow of electrons first in one direction and then in the opposite direction along a wire. A graph of alternating current against time may appear as a sine wave although more complex waveforms, as described in Chapter 13, are also possible. A current which does not have a steady value but in which the electrons move on average in one direction may be described in terms of an AC component added to a DC component, as shown on the right of Fig. 14.1.

The Ampere and Current Measurement

The ampere (A) is the unit of current in the SI system. It represents a flow of 6.24 $\times 10^{18}$ electrons per second past some point, and is defined by means of the electromagnetic force which is associated with an electric current. As mentioned above, whenever an electric current flows in a wire, an associated magnetic field exists around the wire. Moreover, whenever a wire carrying an electric current is placed in a magnetic field, there is a force which tends to move it in a direction perpendicular to both the electric current and the magnetic field.

The interaction of an electric current and a magnetic field is the working principle of instruments such as the galvanometer. In a galvanometer (Fig. 14.2) a coil

Figure 14.2 Principle of the galvanometer

of wire is suspended on jewelled bearings in a magnetic field. The current to be measured passes through this coil and the interaction between the electric current and the magnetic field causes the coil to rotate. The rotational force on the coil is balanced by a hair spring, shown at the bottom of the diagram. The deflection of the coil is proportional to the electric current passing through it and is indicated by a pointer which moves over a scale.

Some recorders used in medical equipment are based on the principle of the galvanometer.

The Electromagnetic Flowmeter

The electromagnetic flowmeter is another example of the application of electro-magnetic effects. If a conductor is moved through a magnetic field, an electric potential develops and the magnitude of this induced potential is proportional to the rate at which the conductor is moved through the magnetic field. As blood is a good conductor of electricity, this principle may be used to measure blood flow.

Consider the artery shown in Fig. 14.3 which lies in a magnetic field produced by the current-carrying coils A and B, the direction of the field being perpendicu-lar to the flow of blood. The blood forms a moving conductor and the potential developed as it flows through the magnetic field is perpendicular to both the direc-tion of flow and the magnetic field, i.e. it is developed across opposite walls of the artery. This potential can be measured by two electrodes, C and D, touching oppo-site sides of the artery.

An electromagnetic flowmeter consists of a C-shaped probe, which contains coils to generate the magnetic field, and two electrodes to measure the potential induced as the blood flows. Although the potential is proportional to the rate at which the blood is flowing, the velocity of the blood varies across the diameter of the blood vessel, so the electromagnetic flowmeter measures an average velocity. It is important that the flowmeter is calibrated with the same type of flow as that which will be present in the vessel on which the measurements are to be made.

In practice, an alternating rather than a steady magnetic field is used and the alternating component of the potential is measured. This improves the accuracy of the measured value.

Figure 14.3 Principle of the electromagnetic blood flowmeter

Current Flow, Energy Production and the Volt

When a current flows, heat and sometimes light energy are produced and the rate at which this energy is produced depends on the circumstances. In the case of an emergency DC-powered operating theatre light, shown in Fig. 14.4, the energy production of heat and light could be 96 watts or 96 joules of energy per second.

In order to drive the electric current through the light bulb, a potential difference must be present across the bulb. The unit of potential difference is the volt, and this is based on the energy production and current flow:

The volt is defined as that potential difference which produces a current of one ampere in a substance when the rate of energy dissipation is one watt.

In other words:

$$\text{Potential difference in volts } V = \frac{\text{Power in watts } W}{\text{Current in amperes } A}$$

In the example shown in Fig. 14.4:

$$\text{Potential difference} = \frac{96 \ W}{4 \ A} = 24 \ V$$

An alternative definition of the volt based on electric charge is sometimes used in connection with the defibrillator, as described later.

Heat Production and AC Units

In addition to its use to define potential, heat production from electric current flow is also used as a basis for comparable AC units of measurement. On the left of Fig. 14.5

Figure 14.4 Example of the definition of potential based on a DC-powered lamp

Figure 14.5 Relationship between an AC and DC supply of equivalent heating effect

is a graph of the potential difference across an item of electric equipment supplied by alternating current. A graph of the current flow would be similar.

Amplitude is normally used as a measure of the size of a sine wave (Chapter 13), but a problem arises in using this simple method in the case of alternating current. An alternating current with a maximum amplitude of one ampere has a smaller heating effect than a constant direct current of one ampere because, in the case of alternating current, the peak flow occurs for only a small fraction of the time. When electricity is used commercially it is the heating and energy production that are of interest. Some units, therefore, are necessary to relate the current and voltage values of AC electricity to the DC units so that the heating effects are the same. The units used are root mean square (rms) values.

An rms voltage of 240 V (the mains potential in the United Kingdom) has an identical heating effect to that of a DC voltage of 240 V when applied across an identical resistor, but its peak voltage is 340 V. The detailed mathematics of rms values are beyond the scope of this book, but Fig. 14.6 illustrates the meaning of the term.

If all the values of the sine wave are squared, all the amplitudes are converted to positive numbers. By taking the mean of these, a value is achieved which is related to the amplitude of the wave. Finally, by taking the square root of this figure, the equivalent DC value is obtained.

Heat Production and Fuses

The rapid increase of heat production with increasing current flow is utilized in the operation of fuses. Essentially, a fuse is a wire of a diameter chosen so that if the current exceeds the rating of the fuse the wire rapidly heats and then melts, so stopping the flow of current. Fuses are incorporated into important circuits in electrical equipment so that if a fault develops, in which a current which is higher than normal flows, the fuse element melts and disconnects the circuit. For the safety of electrical apparatus, it is essential that the correct size of fuse is used.

Electrical Burns

A shock from mains electricity carries a serious risk of ventricular fibrillation (Chapter 16) but sometimes the current only passes through a limb, giving local heating and burns. For example, if a high-voltage source is touched, burns could occur at the fingertip where the current flow is concentrated through a small area. The current flow per unit area is known as current density and the greater the current density, the greater the heating effect.

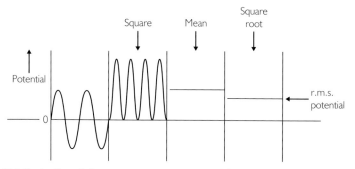

Figure 14.6 Derivation of the root mean square potential

Electrosurgical Equipment

The concept of current density is important because it explains the control of the heating effect of electrosurgical equipment. The passage of direct current or low-frequency alternating current through the body may cause physical sensation, stimulate muscular contraction and give a risk of ventricular fibrillation. These effects become less as the frequency of the current increases, being small above 1 kHz and negligible above 1 MHz, but the heating effect and burning can occur at all frequencies.

Electrosurgical equipment is used to pass a current of a high frequency, typically 1 MHz, through the body in order to cause cutting and coagulation by local heating of body tissues. The degree of heating produced depends on the current density. In electrosurgical equipment, there are two connections to the patient – the neutral or patient plate and the active or cutting electrode used by the surgeon (Fig. 14.7). The same current flows through both connections and, since in the cutting electrode the current is channelled through a very small area, local heating and burning occurs. No burning should occur at the neutral plate, however, as the current flows through a large area.

When monopolar electrosurgical equipment is used, there is normally only one region of high current density – the region adjacent to the active electrode – so this is normally the only region where heating occurs. There are, however, some situations in which current density at other regions in the body can reach a value great enough to cause physical damage. These situations arise when electrosurgical current flows through a cross section of tissue small enough to result in a current density that is sufficiently great to cause burning of tissue or coagulation of blood.

If the neutral plate is not correctly attached to the patient, the area of contact can be reduced to such a degree that burns result where the plate remains in contact with the patient. If the neutral plate becomes completely detached from the patient or is not attached correctly, the current may return to the electrosurgical current generator through any point at which the patient is touching an earthed metal object. In these circumstances, for example, it is possible for a burn to be produced where a patient's hand touches the operating table. Poor neutral plate contact can also result in current flowing through ECG electrodes, causing burns at the sites where they are attached. The likelihood of this happening can be

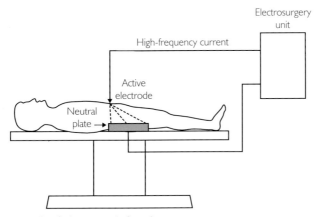

Figure 14.7 Principle of electrosurgical equipment

reduced if the electrodes are applied at sites well away from the place where the active electrode will be used. Electrosurgical current may also take a route that is different from normal if the surgeon activates the electrosurgical unit when the active electrode is not in contact with the patient.

Even in the absence of direct contact, current can flow through capacitance linkage. Because electrosurgery current has a high frequency, capacitance links offer much lower impedance to its flow and such capacitances between the patient and earth or between the patient and the electrosurgery leads give alternative routes for current flow. A thin layer of insulating drapes may not protect the patient from the risk that electrosurgery current could flow and cause a burn.

Current density can reach a hazardous value when the electrosurgical current flows through parts of the body that have small cross sections, such as digits and parts of the ear. Even in regions of the body that have large cross sections, current density can be locally increased if implants of highly conducting materials such as metals are present. The low resistance of the metal compared to the surrounding tissue causes the current to flow preferentially through the implant.

The operation of implanted electromedical devices such as pacemakers can be disrupted if they are exposed to electrosurgical current.

These hazards can often be avoided if an alternative mode of operation of electrosurgical equipment known as bipolar operation is used. Bipolar operation does not require the use of a neutral plate. The electrosurgical current flows through one side of special forceps, through the tissues and back through the other side of the forceps. The current is therefore localized to a small volume of tissue between the tips of the forceps.

Although the use of bipolar electrosurgery would seem to be the solution to the hazards outlined above, the variety of available active electrodes, particularly cutting electrodes, is not as great for bipolar operation as for monopolar operation, so there are some situations in which bipolar operation cannot be used. Bipolar electrosurgery is, however, useful for applications such as neurosurgery, where it is necessary to localize the current and prevent excessive tissue damage.

Properties of Electrical Components

There are standard symbols for electrical components and these are illustrated in Fig. 14.8. The capacitor, inductor and resistor have the properties of capacitance, inductance and resistance, respectively, and these are now considered in more detail.

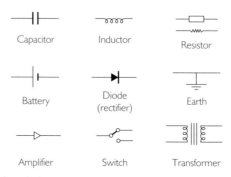

Figure 14.8 Electrical symbols

Capacitance and Electric Charge

Capacitance is a measure of the ability of an object to hold electric charge, charge being a measure of the amount of electricity. The SI unit of charge is the coulomb (C).

The coulomb is the quantity of electric charge which passes some point when a current of one ampere flows for a period of one second:

Coulombs (C) = Amperes (A) × Seconds (s)

The coulomb is an amount of electricity equivalent to 6.24×10^{18} electrons.

The farad is the capacitance of an object for which the electrical potential increases by one volt when one coulomb of charge is added to it:

$$\text{Farads (F)} = \frac{\text{Coulombs (C)}}{\text{Volts (V)}}$$

The Defibrillator

The defibrillator, used for the treatment of ventricular fibrillation, is an example of an instrument in which electric charge is stored and then released in a controlled fashion. The key component for storing the charge is a capacitor (Fig. 14.9), which consists of two plates separated by an insulator. In Fig. 14.9A the defibrillator is at its maximum setting and a potential of 5000 V is applied across the two plates of a capacitor; this produces a store of electrons equivalent to 160 millicoulombs (160 mC) of charge.

The amount of energy stored in a capacitor depends on the charge, the capacitance and the potential.

The energy needed to move an electric charge through a potential difference is

Energy (E) = Potential difference (V) × Charge (Q)

Thus, as the potential difference between the plates of a capacitor increases, more energy is needed to add the same amount of extra charge. The energy, ΔE, needed to add a very small amount of charge, ΔQ, to a capacitor charged to a potential, V, is

$\Delta E = V \Delta Q$

Figure 14.9 Principle of the defibrillator

But the potential difference between the plates changes as the charge is added, since, from the definition of the farad given above,

$$\text{Potential } (V) = \frac{\text{Charge } (Q)}{\text{Capacitance } (C)}$$

So the change in potential produced by adding a small charge ΔQ is

$$\Delta V = \frac{\Delta Q}{C}$$

Therefore

$$\Delta E = C\, V\, \Delta V$$

The total energy stored when many small amounts of energy have been added to the capacitor is calculated by the mathematical process of integration of the above equation:

$$\int dE = C \int V\, dV$$

The result obtained is

$$\text{Stored energy, } E = \tfrac{1}{2}\, CV^2$$

or

$$\text{Stored energy, } E = \tfrac{1}{2}\, QV$$

In the example given:

$$\text{Energy} = \tfrac{1}{2} \times 160 \text{ mC} \times 5000 \text{ V} = 400 \text{ J}$$

To treat a patient in ventricular fibrillation, electrodes are placed on the patient's chest adjacent to the sternum and over the apex of the heart and – by means of switches – the energy stored in the capacitor is released as a current pulse through the patient's chest and heart (Fig. 14.9B). This current pulse, which could be 35 A for 3 ms, gives a synchronous contraction of the myocardium, after which a refractory period and normal or near-normal beats may follow. In practice, an inductor is included in the output circuit of a defibrillator to ensure that the electric pulse has an optimum shape and duration.

When the defibrillator is discharged, the inductor absorbs some of the energy stored in the capacitor so not all of it is delivered to the patient. As it is the energy delivered to the patient that is important in determining the clinical effect, modern defibrillators are calibrated in terms of delivered energy, not stored energy. The maximum delivered energy is normally 360 J. Defibrillators also have a lower maximum setting, normally 100 J, for use with internal cardiac electrodes in a patient with an open chest. Protocols that recommend energy settings for the first and for subsequent shocks exist for both external and internal use of defibrillators.

The working principle described produces a single pulse of current, known as a monophasic waveform, because the current travels in one direction through the chest. There is evidence that the use of two consecutive pulses, in which the current travels first in one direction and then in the other, enables defibrillation to be achieved with a lower energy than with a single pulse. The waveform produced when two pulses are generated in this way is known as a biphasic waveform.

Many defibrillators have provision for synchronized use in treating certain dysrhythmias. When the defibrillator is used in synchronized mode, the energy from the defibrillator must be supplied at the correct time in the cardiac cycle, i.e.

during the R wave. If the pulse is mistimed there is a risk of causing ventricular fibrillation.

Electrostatic Charge

The ability to store a charge is not limited to a capacitor: a charge, usually called an electrostatic charge, can build up on the surface of any object insulated from its surroundings. In the case of a bobbin in a variable orifice flowmeter (Chapter 3), friction may result in electrons being removed from the bobbin surface when it rotates against the wall of the flowmeter. The resulting opposite electric charges on the wall and bobbin can exert a force of attraction leading to the bobbin sticking.

Similarly, insulators may develop charges of this type on their surfaces, with risks of sparks, which can be dangerous in the presence of flammable agents (Chapter 23).

Capacitance and Interference

A capacitor cannot conduct electrons directly across the gap between the plates. Therefore, when direct current is applied to an uncharged capacitor, some current will flow at first to charge up the capacitor plates but will die away as the capacitor becomes fully charged. A capacitor will, however, allow alternating current to pass, as it is continuously being charged and discharged, so allowing current to flow. In anaesthetic practice, this ability of alternating current electricity to pass across an air gap because of capacitance explains why electrical interference may appear on an ECG trace.

Consider the circumstances shown in Fig. 14.10 where an operating theatre light is separated from a patient by an air gap. Mains electricity at a frequency of 50 Hz is passing through the light. The patient on the table, although not directly connected to the light, acts as one plate of a capacitor with the electric light acting as the other plate. A small mains frequency current passes from the lamp to the patient and unfortunately causes a 50 Hz voltage to appear on the ECG trace. This interference may be of sufficient amplitude to obscure the recording.

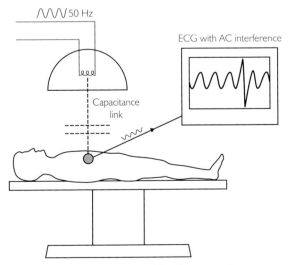

Figure 14.10 Interference on an ECG trace resulting from capacitance

Inductance and Interference

Inductance is based on electromagnetic effects and can also lead to interference in biological electrical signals. An inductor is typically a coil of wire, as indicated by its symbol (see Fig. 14.8). Many components of electrical apparatus have coils of wire with strong magnetic fields around them, e.g. the transformer often found in mains-operated apparatus (Fig. 14.11).

The magnetic field surrounding such apparatus may cause interference in adjacent electrical apparatus and give another source of interference on the ECG trace or on other biological signal displays. In this illustration, the magnetic field formed by the transformer in nearby electrical apparatus induces electric currents in the ECG leads and this source of interference, sometimes called inductive coupling, may lead to interference appearing on the tracing.

Interference from inductive coupling and capacitance effects can be reduced by a system known as screening. The insulated patient monitoring leads are covered by a sheath of woven metal which is earthed, so that interference currents are induced in this metal screen and not in the signal leads. The screening layer is covered by a further layer of insulation.

Signal-to-Noise Ratio

In practice, any electrical waveform or signal includes a certain amount of interference from capacitance and inductance effects and from other sources. This interference is given the term 'noise' from analogy with acoustics, in which noise may be regarded as unwanted sound of various frequencies.

Whether the noise is a practical problem or not depends on its magnitude in relation to the waveform concerned, a useful measure being the signal-to-noise ratio. On the left of Fig. 14.12 is an ECG waveform with a high signal-to-noise ratio, whereas on the right is a similar waveform with a low signal-to-noise ratio. The signal-to-noise ratio is improved if the noise is reduced to a minimum by eliminating its source or by use of differential amplifiers considered in Chapter 15. Unwanted distortion of a biological signal, such as an ECG by electrosurgery, can be avoided by using an electronic filter to cut out the high-frequency electrosurgery signal.

The signal-to-noise ratio cannot be improved by amplifying the waveform because both the signal and the noise will be increased by the same factor, but the

Figure 14.11 Interference on ECG from inductance

Figure 14.12 Signal-to-noise ratio; comparison of high ratio (A) with low ratio (B)

A   B

ratio can be improved by averaging a repetitive waveform, e.g. the signal, over several cycles, and instruments are available to do this electronically. The noise is averaged to zero because of its random nature, whereas the signal remains constant if it is repetitive.

Resistance

The unit of electrical resistance is the ohm (Ω):

The ohm is that resistance which will allow one ampere of current to flow under the influence of a potential of one volt.

$$\text{Resistance } \Omega = \frac{\text{Potential V}}{\text{Current A}}$$

This relationship is known as Ohm's law. Electrical resistance is analogous to flow resistance (Chapter 2), potential taking the place of pressure and current the place of flow. Like flow resistance, electrical resistance varies with the circumstances. A temperature rise increases the resistance of a wire resistor but reduces that of many semiconductors; this fact is used in temperature measurement (Chapter 9) and in the thermal conductivity detector (Chapter 20).

If a wire is stretched it becomes longer and thinner and therefore its resistance increases. Such resistors are known as strain gauges and are used in pressure transducers, as illustrated in Fig. 14.13. In a pressure transducer of this type, movements of the diaphragm with changes of pressure alter the tension in the resistance wire, thus changing its resistance. The changes of current flow through the resistor can then be amplified and displayed as a measure of pressure change.

To monitor or measure such changes of resistance, a circuit known as a Wheatstone bridge is often used. In its original form, this consists of a set of four resistors, a source of electric potential – e.g. a battery – and a galvanometer, arranged as shown in Fig. 14.14. In the example, resistor R_4 could be a strain gauge transducer or a resistance thermometer, whereas R_3 is a variable resistance which can be adjusted until the galvanometer reads zero. In this condition the bridge is said to be balanced and:

$$\frac{R_1}{R_2} = \frac{R_3}{R_4}$$

Figure 14.13 Strain gauge pressure transducer

Pressure →

Strain gauge

Saline

Diaphragm

Figure 14.14 Wheatstone bridge circuit; R_4 is a strain gauge transducer or resistance thermometer and R_3 is a variable resistance which is adjusted until there is a null deflection on the galvanometer

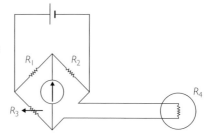

In this form, the Wheatstone bridge is a null deflection system, i.e. no current flows through the galvanometer when the bridge is balanced. In practice, however, the output is amplified and connected to a recorder or oscilloscope in place of the galvanometer and the extent to which the bridge is out of balance is recorded.

Most pressure transducers contain four strain gauges which form the four resistances in the Wheatstone bridge. The transducer is designed so that the resistances of two of the strain gauges at opposite sides of the bridge increase as the pressure increases while the resistances of the other two decrease. This gives a larger potential change at the galvanometer connections of the bridge. The potential is then amplified before it is displayed or recorded.

Figure 14.15 shows another arrangement of resistors R_1–R_5 with a potential V_1 applied across them. If the five resistors are of equal value, by tapping off from point A to one of the other points B, C, D or E, a reduced potential may be obtained and, in the example, potential V_2 is 20% of V_1, i.e. it is attenuated. Sensitivity switches in apparatus may employ a pattern of resistors of this type and in the position shown on the right of the figure, potential V_3 is attenuated to 80% of V_1.

Impedance

The resistance of a resistor to the flow of alternating current does not vary with the frequency of the current. A capacitor can transmit alternating current as mentioned earlier, but in this case high-frequency current passes through it more easily. With an inductor the reverse is true: low-frequency current passes more easily than that of high frequency.

Many circuits and circuit elements behave as though they were made of a combination of resistors, capacitors and inductors and various parts of such circuits possess a particular resistance to the flow of electric current, which in general depends on the frequency of the current flowing. The term impedance is used in preference to resistance when there is a dependence on frequency. The unit of impedance is the same as that of resistance, i.e. the ohm. However, impedance is often indicated by the symbol Z.

Figure 14.15 Principle of an attenuator

Figure 14.16 Effect of impedance at the amplifier Z_A and at the skin and electrodes Z_E on the measurement of a signal potential

A practical example of the use of the variation of impedance with the frequency of the current is the isolating capacitor present in the circuit of some electrosurgical equipment. It offers a high impedance to mains frequency current and so protects the patient from electrocution, and is considered in Chapter 16.

Skin Impedance and Attenuation

An important practical example of impedance occurs in the conduction of a biological electrical signal such as the ECG through the patient's skin to the electrode as, in addition to the resistance at the point of contact, capacitance and inductance may affect the signal. Impedance is less if good contact is maintained at the point where the electrode touches the skin. Many different electrode systems are in use but a typical ECG electrode consists of a metal disc covered with conductive electrode gel and fixed to the patient's skin by a surrounding adhesive flange. The electrode gel reduces the electrical impedance at the point of contact with the skin so that this impedance is as small as possible to avoid attenuation of the signal.

The degree of attenuation of the signal depends not only on the skin impedance but also on the input impedance of the monitoring apparatus used to detect it.

Study of Fig. 14.16 and comparison with Fig. 14.15 illustrates the principle. On the left of Fig. 14.16 is an example in which there is a high impedance Z_E from the skin and electrodes. This could arise from dried electrode gel or a loose electrode contact. In addition, there is a relatively low amplifier input impedance Z_A. The signal is greatly attenuated because of the ratio of the two impedances Z_E and Z_A.

The diagram on the right of Fig. 14.16 shows an amplifier with a high input impedance used with electrodes with good skin contact to give negligible attenuation of the input signal. Most amplifiers now have a very high input impedance to allow satisfactory ECG recordings even with the simpler and smaller skin electrodes. A high amplifier input impedance also protects the patient against electrocution (Chapter 16).

Skin impedance is lowered when the skin is moist. The degree of moisture depends on sympathetic tone, so skin impedance has been used as a measure of the autonomic activity. This test is known as the galvanic skin response, or GSR.

Biological Electrical Potentials: Their Display and Recording

15

Origin of Biological Potentials

The membrane of a cell is composed of phospholipids and has a sandwich structure, with a hydrophobic fatty interior and a protein–carbohydrate exterior. The metabolic mechanisms pump sodium ions out of the cell, and potassium ions in through the cell membrane. These ions carry electric charges, so that the net result is a positive charge of around 90 mV at the exterior compared with the interior of the cell.

As shown in Fig. 15.1, a rapid loss of this potential takes place prior to the contraction of cardiac or skeletal muscle. During this period of depolarization, sodium ions move into the cell and potassium ions move out through the membrane. Finally, the membrane recovers its potential as the sodium–potassium pump restores the status quo. Other ion movements also occur. In cardiac muscle, for example, calcium ions as well as sodium ions enter the cell, so maintaining a longer period of depolarization than that in the skeletal muscle. Adjacent areas of membrane are destabilized by the region of depolarization and undergo the same changes, so that a wave of depolarization spreads over the muscle. Similar changes take place at the surface membrane of a neurone to propagate the nerve impulse.

These waves of electric potential change are transmitted through the tissues overlying the nerves and muscles. The signal can be detected by suitable electrodes placed on the skin and displayed as an electroencephalogram (EEG), electrocardiogram (ECG) or electromyogram (EMG). The graphs obtained of voltage against time are complex wave patterns and these waves may be separated into a collection of pure sine waves by Fourier analysis, as described in Chapter 13.

Electrocardiogram

During a cardiac cycle, a wave of depolarization passes from the atrial pacemaker cells over the atrium and down the AV bundle to spread through the ventricular myocardial syncytium. Potentials from the heart are transmitted through the tissues and can be detected by electrodes to give an ECG recording. These potentials are attenuated as the signal passes through the tissues. Hence the size of the ECG signal detected is only 1–2 mV instead of the original potential of about 90 mV mentioned above. The larger the bulk of the cardiac muscle through which the waves of depolarization pass, the larger the potential detected at the surface, so there is a large QRS complex from the depolarization wave in the ventricles and a smaller P wave from the atria.

The actual appearance of the ECG depends on the position of the electrodes relative to the heart (Fig. 15.2). Because the atrial signal spreads outwards, the P wave is usually positive regardless of the electrode position. However, in the case of the ventricles the wave of depolarization travels downwards and to the left, so

Figure 15.1 Depolarization changes at a cell membrane

Figure 15.2 The ECG signal picked up by electrodes at A differs from that at B because it depends on the position of the electrodes relative to the wave of depolarization spreading through the cardiac muscle

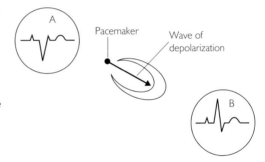

the QRS complexes vary in appearance according to the electrode position. With an oesophageal electrode positioned close behind the atria of the heart, a particularly clear ECG signal of the P waves is obtainable. The time intervals in the complexes are important. For example, a PR interval of over 200 ms indicates delayed conduction from the atria.

Because other muscles give rise to potentials, the patient must relax and make no movement during the recording.

Electromyogram

The electromyogram or EMG records muscle potentials either from surface electrodes or from needle electrodes in the muscle itself. The potentials detected range from about 100 µV to many mV. Skeletal muscle potentials differ from those of the ECG in that they have a much shorter duration, perhaps 5–10 ms, so the EMG gives sharp spikes in place of the complex ECG pattern. The short duration arises because skeletal muscle repolarizes more rapidly than cardiac muscle and has cells which do not polarize in synchrony with adjoining cells. As shown in Fig. 15.3, the amplitude of the EMG signal spike depends upon the number of muscle fibres simultaneously stimulated. This, in turn, depends upon the number of fibres stimulated by the motor neurone. At the top of the figure, each motor neurone supplies about eight muscle fibres (for example, in an eye muscle), and so a small spike

Figure 15.3 EMG potentials from an impulse from the motor neurone supplying an eye muscle (A) and a limb muscle (B)

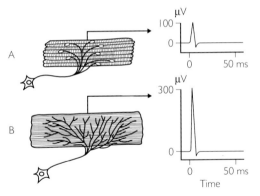

potential occurs. Figure 15.3B illustrates a limb muscle with a motor unit of 200 fibres, so a larger spike potential results.

Electroencephalogram

In the electroencephalogram, the EEG, 16 electrodes are positioned around the patient's head to pick up the characteristic potentials from the nerve tracts, brain-stem and cerebrum. The potentials are much smaller than those of the ECG, being only about 50 μV.

The appearance of the EEG wave pattern is also important. For example, slow, low-frequency waves may indicate cerebral hypoxia. In anaesthesia, increasing depth of anaesthesia is usually accompanied by a decrease in the frequency and amplitude of the EEG. Because the standard EEG is too complex for routine use in anaesthesia, alternative techniques have been developed. These techniques are considered in Chapter 26.

Range of Frequencies and Potentials

The relevant ranges of frequencies and potentials of biological signals are shown in Fig. 15.4. In the ECG, the frequency range is about 0.5–100 Hz, whereas in an

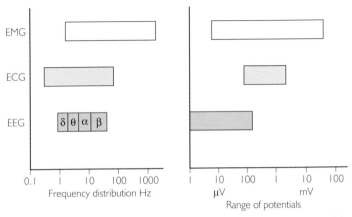

Figure 15.4 Range of frequencies and potentials for biological electrical potentials

EEG, the frequency distribution is smaller. The beta waves of the EEG are in the range of 15–60 Hz and the slow delta waves start at about 1 Hz. In an EMG, there are sharp spikes indicating that an analysis of the waveform would result in a very large frequency distribution of sine waves.

The Black Box Concept

When recording biological variables, the amplifier, recorder and input transducer, if required, may be regarded as a series of black boxes, as indicated in Fig. 15.5. By simplifying the processes of detection, amplification and recording of biological signals in this way, it becomes unnecessary to understand the complicated interactions of individual electrical components in the system. What is essential is to ensure that the electrical characteristics of the signal from the output of any one black box, such as voltage, current and frequency range, are compatible with the input of the next black box in the system. Provided that they are matched, the black boxes can be connected together to provide a satisfactory monitoring system.

In modern apparatus, components are miniaturized and thus the whole of an amplifier black box becomes a small item incorporated in the recording or display system. An input transducer is needed for arterial or venous pressure measurement or for temperature measurement, but electrodes are used to pick up biological electrical potentials directly.

Electrodes

Problems can arise at the junction between the skin surface and the electrodes used to measure biological electrical potentials. The combination of the metal electrode, the gel used to form an electrical contact between the metal and the skin, and the electrolytes present in the skin and tissues form an electric cell which generates a potential. This electrode potential and the impedance between the electrode and the skin may change if the electrode moves. The biological electrical potential itself causes a small current to flow through the electrode and this current alters the distribution of ions at the interface between the metal and electrolyte in the electrode.

Figure 15.5 Black box concept

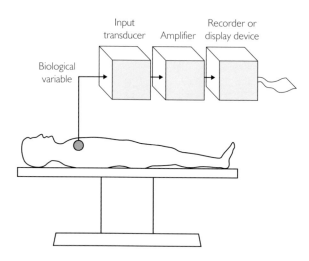

Figure 15.6 Problems at
skin–electrode junction

Chemical changes
Potential generated
Variable impedance

Electrode

Skin

This in turn alters the electrode potential, an effect known as polarization. Alterations in the electrode potential are recorded by the signal display system in addition to the biological electrical potentials themselves.

An extreme example of polarization may arise when a defibrillator is used. The high current flow through the defibrillator electrodes can polarize them severely, so direct recording of the ECG from these electrodes may temporarily cease after defibrillation.

These problems can be reduced by the choice of a suitable electrode. Use of a silver electrode in contact with silver chloride on its surface, which is, in turn, in contact with chloride ions in a gel solution in a sponge pad secured to the skin, results in a fairly stable electrode potential that does not interfere with recording. The electrode and pad are securely fixed to the skin with an adhesive disc.

Amplifiers

These are usually differential amplifiers, and measure the difference between the potential from two sources, indicated as S_1 and S_2 in Fig. 15.7. The advantage of this system is that any interference which is common to the input terminals, such as that from 50 Hz mains, is eliminated, as only the difference between the terminals is amplified in the differential amplifier. The ability of the differential amplifier to reject the interference common to both electrodes is known as the common-mode rejection ratio. All biopotential amplifiers require good common-

S_1 50 Hz
S_2 50 Hz

Figure 15.7 Differential amplifier

mode rejection because biopotentials are often small in comparison to sources of interference.

In the case of the ECG, several electrode connections are used with a switch so the potential difference between appropriate electrodes may be displayed. One of the electrodes is used as a reference potential for the ECG amplifier (Chapter 16).

Amplifiers contain some components that are made from semiconductor material. It has already been pointed out that the resistance of semiconductors varies with temperature; hence changes in environmental temperature may cause the DC potential at the output of an amplifier to change, although the DC potential at the input is constant. The problem is known as drift and is much less serious if an amplifier is designed only for AC potentials.

The amplifier for a particular biological signal must be able to respond to the range of frequencies concerned (see Fig. 15.4). The range of frequencies over which the amplification is relatively constant is known as the bandwidth of the amplifier. Interference in the signal may be avoided if the bandwidth of the equipment used is selected to match the signal correctly. For example, if the upper limit of the amplifier frequency range is chosen correctly when EEG potentials are being recorded, interference from higher-frequency muscle potentials may be avoided.

The amplifier must also be suitable for the voltage range of the signal. Thus, a particularly sensitive amplifier is needed for EEG measurement as the size of the signal is so small, perhaps 50 µV, compared with the ECG signal of about 1 mV. The ratio of the voltage at the output of an amplifier to the signal voltage at the input is known as the gain of the amplifier. Both the gain of an amplifier and the common-mode rejection ratio are typically measured on a logarithmic scale with a unit known as the bel. However, the decibel (dB), i.e. one-tenth of a bel, is normally used in place of the bel, as it is a more convenient unit. The ratio of two voltages, V_1 and V_2, is expressed in decibels as follows:

$$\text{Voltage ratio} = 20 \log_{10} \frac{V_1}{V_2} \text{ decibels}$$

The decibel is also used as a unit of measurement in sound, where it is used to compare the power of the sound being measured to that which would be present at the threshold of hearing.

The Initiation of Electrical Potentials

In addition to the detection of biological potentials, electrical apparatus is often used to provide an electrical stimulus. One example is the use of the defibrillator considered in Chapter 14. Other examples are pacemakers used to maintain cardiac rhythm, nerve stimulators used in studies of neuromuscular contraction and stimulators used in the treatment of chronic pain conditions. A square-wave electrical pulse is used in these cases and the potentials and frequencies depend on the circumstances.

The Cardiac Pacemaker

The stimulating electrode may be inserted into the right ventricle of the heart by cardiac catheterization or by embedding it in the muscle of the ventricle. The potentials are up to 4 V, and the frequency of the signal is adjusted according to the heart rate required. The duration of the pulse is under 1 ms. Pacemakers and their safety aspects are considered further in Chapter 16.

The Nerve Stimulator

A nerve stimulator produces electrical pulses to stimulate motor or sensory nerves. In the motor nerve stimulator used to assess neuromuscular block, two small pre-gelled silver/silver chloride pad electrodes are applied. The negative electrode, in this case called the active electrode, is placed over the ulnar nerve at the wrist (Fig. 15.8), with the positive electrode a few centimetres proximal. These electrodes give good electrical contact, having a skin–electrode impedance of perhaps 1 kΩ. The stimulator gives a very short electrical pulse of about 200 µs, with a peak current of up to 60 mA.

Following each pulse, thumb and finger movement are seen and can be assessed by the strength of the thumb movement measured by palpation or by a strain gauge. The current is adjusted to that needed to give a maximal muscle contraction. A train of four pulses can be given at a frequency of 2 Hz (so that the four pulses cover 2 seconds), and this technique has been found useful to assess the type and degree of nerve block. In partial non-depolarizing block, for example, the strength of the thumb movement fades over the four pulses, whereas in complete block, all four twitches in the train are absent. Instead of the train-of-four technique, tetanic stimulation at a frequency of 50 Hz can be used, but this is painful for a conscious patient.

Electrical Stimulators in Pain Treatment

Much chronic pain is transmitted by small afferent fibres. One theory suggests that stimulation by larger afferents inhibits transmission or 'closes the gate' on the transmission of pain from the smaller fibres. This effect may take place in the spinal cord and be potentiated by the production of pharmacologically active substances, i.e. endorphins, in the central nervous system in response to stimulation of the larger afferent fibres.

Electrical stimulation of these fibres may be by skin electrodes, nerve stimulation or direct stimulation from electrodes implanted over the dorsal columns of the spinal cord. The stimulator used with electrodes on the skin is sometimes called TNS or TENS (transcutaneous electrical nerve stimulation). The TENS apparatus has small conductive electrode pads to which gel is applied before fixing to the skin.

As in the case of the stimulator used to assess neuromuscular block, the currents used in the TENS stimulator are up to 60 mA, and the pulse durations are also comparable, being between 60 and 380 µs. The pulse frequency is 2–200 Hz, depending upon the stimulator and the clinical requirements. When in use, the patient feels a sensation of tingling and warmth.

Figure 15.8 Use of the train of four pulses from a nerve stimulator

Stimulator

Thumb movement

The effectiveness of electrical stimulators varies greatly with different patients. Consequently, a patient must adjust the controls of the stimulator to provide the pulse amplitude, width and repetition frequency that gives the best pain relief. This should be done under medical supervision as misuse may result in tissue damage.

In addition to the use of nerve stimulators for pain relief, some anaesthetists use them as an aid to identify nerves prior to the administration of local analgesics.

Pain is a subjective sensation; two techniques are commonly used to assess it. One is the ordered category scale in which the patient is asked to quantify the pain experienced according to a scale such as 1 = no pain, 2 = mild pain, 3 = moderate pain and 4 = severe pain. An alternative technique is the visual analogue scale (VAS). The patient is presented with a 100 mm-long horizontal line marked on a paper. The extreme left of the line represents no pain, whereas the extreme right-hand end represents the worst pain imaginable. Patients are asked to quantify their pain by marking the 100 mm line at a point equivalent to their perception of the pain.

Electroconvulsive Therapy

Another type of stimulator is that used for electroconvulsive therapy, ECT, in the treatment of some psychiatric illnesses. Two-saline soaked pads are applied, one to each temple of the anaesthetized patient, and a current of perhaps 850 mA is passed through the brain to induce a major cerebral seizure. The recommended stimulation is in the form of brief pulses of 1.25 ms repeated 26 times a second, i.e. 26 Hz, for a total time of 2–5 seconds. The potential will depend on the impedance between the electrodes, but could be about 250 V.

Signal Display

There are several ways in which biological electrical potentials from patients can be displayed. If the signal from a patient is steady or slowly changing then an analogue display in which a lever moves over a scale can provide a clear visual indication of the size of a variable. A digital meter works by means of integrated circuits (Chapter 25) and displays values as a set of figures. This can be an advantage when figures are to be noted, and a digital display may also be more accurate and easier to read at a distance. Nevertheless, it is difficult to observe trends on a digital meter. Biological potentials change rapidly, so some form of recording on paper or the use of an oscilloscope screen may be more suitable than a meter in these cases.

The galvanometer, discussed in Chapter 14, is the basis of the usual type of analogue meter. This type of analogue meter has several shortcomings however, so it has been superseded as a display device in most items of medical equipment. On its own, it provides no permanent record, and the inertia of its coil and needle precludes the display of rapidly changing signals.

Galvanometer Recorders

The galvanometer can be modified to provide a continuous record: one method is to conduct ink through a capillary to a writing point at the end of the galvanometer needle, as shown in Fig. 15.9. An alternative method uses a galvanometer needle with a heated tip so that a record may be produced on heat-sensitive paper, as illustrated in Fig. 15.10.

Figure 15.9 Galvanometer
recorder

Figure 15.10 Heated stylus
recorder

Heated stylus

Heat-sensitive paper

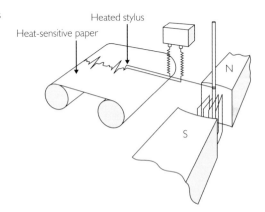

In these recorders the inertia of the galvanometer needle is increased by the heated stylus tip or by the capillary tube carrying ink. Thus, the speed at which the needle will respond to the signal is limited. These recorders cannot therefore be used to display a rapidly changing signal such as the EMG. In the case of the heated stylus recorder illustrated, the maximum frequency response is about 80 Hz and is just adequate to cope with the recording of an ECG for clinical purposes.

The total inertia of the moving parts may be reduced if the tracing arm is replaced by a jet of ink, as illustrated in Fig. 15.11. The frequency response of such a system increases from the 80 Hz of the heated stylus type of recorder to about 500 Hz. But the disadvantages of such a recorder are the increased cost and the need for greater care in use to avoid blockage of the ink jets.

Another problem which can arise in the simpler recorders is related to the fact that the writing point traces an arc (Fig. 15.12). Inaccuracies can arise when measuring the deflection in this case. It is the angle, or arc, through which the pen moves that measures the potential applied to the galvanometer, and the linear deflection of the trace is not directly proportional to the length of the arc.

The relationship is indicated in Fig. 15.12. If H is the deflection of the recorder point measured at right angles from the base line, H is $r \sin A$, where r is the length of the recorder pointer and A the angle of deflection. If angle A is measured in radians, arc length S is equal to $r \times A$. Then the error is as follows:

Figure 15.11 Ink jet recorder

Figure 15.12 Sine distortion

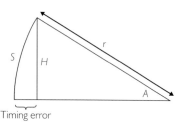

$$\text{Error} = H - S = r\,(\sin A - A)$$

Sine distortion would be less if the radius r of the arm of the recorder were increased. However, it is not practical to have a long arm in a simple recorder as this increases inertia.

In addition to sine distortion, there is also a timing error in the direction in which the paper moves (as shown in the figure), and this is related to the cosine of angle A.

With some recorders, the grid on the paper has a curved vertical axis. This helps to compensate visually for the fact that the recorder traces an arc, and solves the problem of the timing error (Fig. 15.13). If the calibration of the grid is appropriately nonlinear, this can compensate for sine distortion.

In the case of the heated stylus recorder, this arcing may be corrected by replacing the recorder point with a heated rod system, as illustrated in Fig. 15.14. The rod rides over the curved surface of the paper, so that vertical lines are straight.

In the ink jet recorder, the jet strikes the vertical surface of the recording paper and this removes the curvature in the tracing.

Figure 15.13 Arc distortion of tracing

Figure 15.14 Use of a ridge on recording paper to remove arc distortion

Heated stylus over ridge

These systems remove both the grosser curvature and the horizontal timing error which are present with the simpler recorders. Nevertheless, there is still a slight error, known as tangent distortion, when the height of the tracing is used as a measure of the deflection because this height is not directly proportional to the angle of the deflection.

In these cases, as illustrated in Fig. 15.15, the effective length of the recorder pointer R varies with the movement of the galvanometer during recording. The distance of the tracing paper from the pivot of the galvanometer is a constant D, and arc S represents the true deflection of the galvanometer angle A caused by the signal. If A is in radians, the error is as follows:

$$\text{Error} = H - S = D \,(\tan A - A)$$

Like sine distortion, tangent distortion is less when angle A is smaller.

Potentiometric Recorders

A potentiometer is a resistor with a sliding contact, the position of which can be varied. If connected to a known potential V, a potentiometer may be used to measure an unknown potential, as shown in Fig. 15.16. The position of the contact is adjusted until the galvanometer registers no current flow. Under this condition, if the distance of the contact is d along a resistance with total length l, then:

$$\text{Unknown voltage} = V \times \frac{d}{l}$$

Figure 15.17 indicates how the potentiometric recorder is based on the principle of the potentiometer. The sliding contact C follows the signal potential but,

Figure 15.15 Tangent distortion

Figure 15.16 Potentiometer

Figure 15.17 Potentiometric recorder

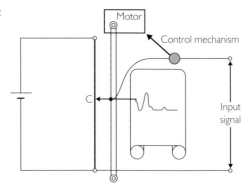

instead of being adjusted manually, it is moved by an electric motor. The motor is driven by an amplifier, which measures the difference between the signal potential and the potential at C. This is done in such a way that point C is always returned to a position in the potentiometer where the potential is equal to the input potential; a writing stylus is added to trace the movement of contact C on a chart as shown.

A motor moving a pointer containing ink over a wide chart cannot respond rapidly to sudden changes, so potentiometric recorders have a limited frequency response. They may be used for longer-term recordings, such as the patient's temperature, and, in contrast to the narrower tracings usual with galvanometer recorders, a potentiometric recorder can provide a wide tracing with an ink pen system and can also permit overlapping tracings.

If several simultaneous tracings are required, then a number of amplifiers and motors are needed to drive pens with different coloured inks over the chart. There is then the difficulty that the recordings are offset in time from each other, i.e. their positions on the chart are staggered because space is needed for each moving stylus. However, chart recorders are available in which the input signal for each channel is stored electronically and its timing adjusted, so that recordings are produced in synchrony although the pen positions are staggered.

Thermal Array Printers

The printing head in a thermal array printer contains a row of very small elements, each of which can be heated under electronic control by the passage of an electric current through it. The paper used to produce the recording contains a coloured layer underneath a white layer. As the paper passes over the print head, the appropriate elements are heated. The heated elements remove the white top layer of the paper, allowing the coloured layer underneath to be seen and producing the required waveform on the paper. The system can also be used to produce alphanumerics and graticules on the paper.

As thermal array printers do not suffer from inertia or distortion, they overcome most of the problems associated with the types of recorder considered so far and have largely superseded other recorders in the type of equipment that most anaesthetists use.

Display of High-Frequency Signals

A signal such as the electromyogram is composed of a mixture of frequencies, the highest of which are many kilohertz. A chart recorder is not capable of displaying such high-frequency signals directly, but a technique is available to store the signal electronically and then display it at a later time. The technique involves the conversion of an analogue signal into digital form for subsequent storage, the process taking place at very high speed. Once the signal is stored, it is available for further processing as required. This may include tracing the recording onto a chart recorder at a slower speed than it was initially acquired or displaying the signal on an oscilloscope.

The Cathode Ray Tube

The principle of the cathode ray tube (CRT) is illustrated in Fig. 15.18. A hot cathode produces an electron beam which passes through two deflecting devices, one of which deflects the beam horizontally on the X axis and the other vertically on the Y axis. In the case illustrated, these are in the form of simple plates which deflect the beam, depending on the potential applied to them. The beam then strikes a fluorescent screen where it produces a tracing. The advantage of the cathode ray tube is that the electron beam has negligible inertia, thus leading to a very high frequency response.

Cathode ray tubes form part of medical monitoring and display equipment. In many applications, a sawtooth potential deflects the beam in the X direction. The signal, which may be any biological electrical potential such as an ECG or perhaps a blood pressure tracing from an arterial pressure transducer and which has been processed as described below, deflects the beam in the Y direction. For an ECG, the sensitivity control of the oscilloscope is usually adjusted so that a 1 mV calibration signal gives 1 cm vertical displacement of the trace, while the speed

Figure 15.18 Cathode ray tube

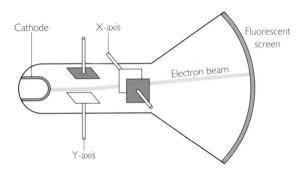

control alters the frequency of the sawtooth potential and so controls the time taken for one horizontal sweep of the trace.

In patient monitoring equipment, the incoming electrical signal is normally divided as it arrives into fragments of a few milliseconds duration, resulting in a series of discrete values. These are stored electronically in a memory bank in digital form. The complete memory store is continually scanned and displayed on the screen. As new fragments of information are added at one end of the memory, old fragments are removed from the other end. At any instant the input of new information to the memory can be stopped, and the contents of the store when read out repeatedly on the screen produce a frozen trace. As a result of the digitization process, the frequency response of the complete monitor is somewhat less than that of the cathode ray tube itself, though still fully adequate for ECG monitoring, for example.

Monitoring equipment uses integrated circuits to process the signal prior to its display and may therefore show additional relevant data in the form of a digital readout on the screen. Thus, analysis of the frequency of the QRS complexes of the ECG gives pulse rate, and analysis of the arterial pressure waveform can give systolic, mean and diastolic pressures. For observation of several tracings and figures simultaneously, colour tracings and figures may be provided.

Many monitors are capable of being coupled to computers and recorders to provide a printed copy of the data. Alternatively, a record can be stored on a magnetic disk for subsequent analysis.

Electrical Safety

16

When the flow of electric current through a person is excessive, there is a risk of electric shock and burns. Burns resulting from the flow of electric current are discussed in Chapter 14. Electric shock and its prevention are considered in this chapter.

Mains Supply, Skin Impedance and Earth

In order to understand how the risk of electric shock can arise, consider how electricity is supplied to a hospital (Fig. 16.1). A power station supplies electricity at very high voltage to a substation, where the voltage is reduced by a transformer. The current passes between the substation and the hospital along two wires, the live and the neutral, the neutral wire being connected to earth at the substation. Mains electric sockets in the hospital provide connections to the live and neutral conductors and also to a third conductor, which is connected to earth at the hospital.

If a person touches the live wire in the hospital, an electric circuit can be completed through the body, through the earth, and back to the substation. This could be an anaesthetist touching the live wire in a damaged cable as shown in the figure, so that current passes through the anaesthetist and through the antistatic footwear to the earthed antistatic floor. The effect of the electric shock received by the anaesthetist depends on the size of the current which flows. If this is only a small current of 1 mA, the anaesthetist is likely to feel a tingling sensation on touching the live parts of the apparatus, but he will suffer no serious effects. The mains electricity supply in the United Kingdom is at 240 V potential (in North America and some other countries it is 110 V) and the current which flows through the anaesthetist depends on the impedance presented to this flow. In the situation described, the impedance of the skin and tissues may be ignored as this is small compared to that of the antistatic footwear and floor. If the impedance of the footwear and the antistatic floor is 240 kΩ, the current is 1 mA, i.e.

$$\text{Current} = \frac{\text{Potential}}{\text{Impedance}} = \frac{240}{240,000} \times 1000 \text{ mA} = 1 \text{ mA}$$

Antistatic shoes have a strong protective effect by virtue of their high resistance. It is recommended that the impedance of such shoes should be between 75 kΩ and 10 MΩ when new. This value of impedance is low enough to permit safe dissipation of electrostatic charges, but high enough to give some protection against electric shock.

In Fig. 16.2, the anaesthetist is touching faulty apparatus but is wearing non-standard footwear, and is standing in a pool of saline which he has spilt on the floor and which is in contact with an earthed water pipe. Saline is a good conductor of electricity and so in these circumstances a higher current flows. As the current increases over 1 mA, the sensation of tingling gives way to pain and the current stimulates muscular contraction. In the case illustrated, the current could be 24 mA and the anaes-

Figure 16.1 Power supply to the hospital and the position of the anaesthetist in completing the circuit between the live wire and earth

thetist would be unable to release the handle of the electrically faulty apparatus. The current therefore, continues to flow, passing to earth through the anaesthetist's body, the footwear, the pool of saline and the water pipe. In these circumstances, current need pass through the chest for only a fraction of a second before ectopic beats occur, with the risk of ventricular fibrillation, a risk which increases as the current increases. In this case, the impedance of the footwear is negligible and the impedance of the floor has been bypassed. The internal tissue impedance of the anaesthetist, too, is small, being only a few hundred ohms. Most of the impedance now occurs at the points of contact with the skin, i.e. the hand with the equipment and the feet with the shoes. In other words, the skin impedance is the main component, being perhaps a few kilohms. If it is 10 kΩ, the current may be calculated as before, i.e.:

$$\text{Current} = \frac{\text{Potential}}{\text{Impedance}} = \frac{240}{10,000} \times 1000 \text{ mA} = 24 \text{ mA}$$

Skin impedance is not constant, however, but depends on many factors. If the anaesthetist's hands are wet, and if the surface area of the hand touching the live

Figure 16.2 Increased risk to an anaesthetist wearing nonstandard footwear in a pool of saline

equipment is large, the impedance may be much less than 10 kΩ and the current proportionally greater.

The impedances of the contacts with the source of electric current and with the earth are of vital importance when considering the risk of ventricular fibrillation in equipment users and patients. As mentioned above, the skin impedance is not a constant factor. Thus, the impedance is high with dry skin, lower if the skin is damp, and it is lowered further if there are needles or cannulae passing through the skin. Finally, the larger the area of contact with the source of electricity or with the earth, the lower is the impedance.

The risk of ventricular fibrillation is affected by additional factors such as the timing of current flowing through the heart. The risk is much greater if the electric current passes through the heart during the repolarization of the muscle cells, which occurs during the early T wave of the ECG. Another factor is the form of the electric current. Mains alternating current of 50 Hz is more dangerous than high-frequency current of 1 kHz or greater. Finally, ventricular fibrillation from electric shock can occur at a lower current in patients with myocardial disease or dysrhythmias.

Protection Against Electric Shock

The risk of electric shock can be greatly reduced if equipment is constructed and maintained to a suitable standard. All medical equipment purchased in the UK, used in the patient environment and affecting patient safety, should meet the requirements of British Standard EN 60601: Safety of Medical Electrical Equipment. The corresponding international standard is International Electrotechnical Commission Standard 601.

These standards include the classification of equipment according to the means of protection it provides against electric shock arising from contact with the mains electricity supply. There are three classes for electromedical equipment.

Class I Equipment

In class I equipment, any conducting part that is accessible to the user, such as the metal case of an instrument, is connected to an earth wire, which becomes the third wire connected via the plug to the mains supply socket (Fig. 16.3). If a fault occurs in the equipment in which a connection is made inadvertently between the live supply and the case of the equipment, a circuit is completed from the power source, through the case of the instrument and then to earth, so that a high current flows which melts a protecting fuse (or fuses). This disconnects the circuit and removes the live potential from the equipment case.

For this protective system to operate the earth wire must be connected correctly and fuses must be present in the live and neutral wires. In the UK, a fuse is also incorporated in the mains plug.

Class II Equipment

In class II equipment, also called double-insulated equipment, all accessible parts are protected by two layers of insulation, or by a single layer of reinforced insulation, so that there is no possibility of a person touching any conducting part that may become live through the occurrence of a single fault. An earth wire is not required for class II equipment.

Figure 16.3 Class 1 equipment: principle of earthing of the metal case of apparatus and the use of a fuse

Internally Powered Equipment

The third class of equipment is known as internally powered equipment and has its own power source, such as batteries, located within the equipment. Although the risk of electric shock may still be present, the particular risks associated with the use of mains electricity are avoided.

Shock Risks with Earthed Equipment

A patient who is allowed to come into contact with earthed equipment of class I may be at risk of electrocution under some circumstances. Figure 16.4 shows a patient in theatre, whose feet have been allowed to touch the stem of a portable lamp, the outside of which is earthed. It provides a direct route through the patient from faulty live apparatus to earth, the only protection being the size of the patient's skin impedance. If the latter is 10 kΩ, the current through the chest will be 24 mA, which is capable of causing ventricular fibrillation.

Space blankets are made of metal-coated plastic and may constitute an electrical hazard if they come into contact with earthed metal apparatus, thus forming

Figure 16.4 Risk of electrocution of a patient in contact with earthed equipment

a low resistance path to earth. These blankets are used to reduce hypothermia by reflecting radiant heat back to the patient but they must not be used in theatre, especially if electrosurgical equipment is in use, because of the electrical safety hazard and also because they can burn. In intensive care areas and in proximity to monitoring equipment, they should be used only with care.

Patient electrodes, used for example with ECG apparatus and electrosurgical equipment, may provide a path for current to flow to earth under faulty conditions with the associated risk of electric shock.

As described in Chapter 14, the alternating current of mains electricity can produce small currents and potentials by inductive and capacitive coupling. These currents can be induced in the metal case of an instrument, in other circuits or even in a person touching insulated equipment. Such currents, known as leakage currents, will not cause gross electric shock but in some circumstances they can give rise to the danger known as microshock.

Microshock

Ventricular fibrillation resulting from electric shock is caused by the passage of an electric current through the myocardium. If the electric current passes from a hand to the feet (see Fig. 16.4), it not only passes through the heart but also through a portion of the trunk. Therefore, the total current flow through the heart itself is only a fraction of the 24 mA which may pass from the hand to the feet. It is the fraction of the current passing through the myocardium or the current density (current per unit area) in the region of the myocardium that determines whether ventricular fibrillation will occur.

If there is a faulty intracardiac catheter passing from an item of monitoring equipment into the heart itself (Fig. 16.5) and if this catheter touches the wall of the heart, any electric current flowing along the catheter will pass through a very small area of the heart. In such a case, a current of only 150 μA may produce the same current density in a portion of the myocardium as that produced by 24 mA flowing from a hand to the feet. Hence, ventricular fibrillation may be induced. This is the phenomenon known as microshock.

As with gross electric shock, the severity of microshock increases as the frequency of the current decreases, so the risk is greatest at low frequencies such as mains frequency and with direct current.

Note that it is not necessary for the faulty apparatus to be at mains potential for there to be a risk of microshock. As microshock currents have values of microamperes rather than milliamperes, the potentials can be proportionately scaled down and there is a risk of microshock from a potential lower than even 1 V. In the case illustrated in Fig. 16.5, equipment attached to the catheter is faulty and a small leakage current is flowing through the catheter and through the heart in the earthed patient. In the illustration, the patient is earthed by his feet being in contact with a metal lamp but, alternatively, he might be earthed by contact through the operating table or through faulty equipment. Although the impedance to earth through these items may be high enough to protect against major electric shock, this may not prevent the flow of a small current giving the risk of microshock.

The anaesthetist too may act as an earthing point for the patient if in contact simultaneously with the earthed casing of apparatus and with the patient (Fig. 16.6). In this event, the small current from the faulty equipment travels via the cardiac catheter to give a risk of microshock in the patient, even though the current flowing through the anaesthetist is too small to be noticed by him.

Figure 16.5 Risk of microshock

Microshock is a risk in patients who are fitted with an intracardiac pacemaker with an external lead. A temperature-monitoring probe placed in the lower third of the oesophagus behind the left atrium also gives a possible route for electricity to pass in close proximity to the heart, although it may not be as dangerous as a catheter placed directly in the cavities of the heart.

Isolated Patient Circuits

Some equipment, for example monitoring equipment, requires electrical connections to be made to the patient. In order to obtain a good connection, a deliberate effort is made to reduce the impedance at the junction between the electrode and the skin. This decreases the protection that the skin might otherwise have provided in reducing the risk of electric shock.

To counteract this problem, most equipment that requires electrical connections to be made to a patient uses an isolated patient circuit, also known as a floating circuit. The electrical circuit of the equipment is divided into two parts: a mains part, which contains a power supply driven directly by the mains; and an isolated part, which is separated from the mains part by an electrical barrier

Figure 16.6 Anaesthetist as a potential earthing point for the patient

intended to provide protection should a fault develop in the mains part and to reduce the flow of mains leakage currents in the patient circuit.

Leakage Current Standards

In addition to the division of equipment into three classes according to the means adopted to provide protection against the hazard of electric shock from the mains electricity supply, electromedical equipment is classified according to the maximum leakage currents permissible for particular applications. Exacting standards have been defined which are based upon assessments on equipment when operated with faults such as reversal of the neutral and live wires or disconnection of the earth wire.

Equipment used with electrodes which may contact the heart directly is termed type CF, indicating that it is for cardiac use and has a floating circuit. In this case, the leakage current through its intracardiac connection must be under 50 μA, even if it is operating with a single fault.

Other medical monitoring equipment is termed type B, or type BF if it has a floating circuit. For these types of equipment, the maximum permitted patient leakage current is higher than for CF equipment, being 500 μA under single-fault conditions.

The values of the maximum permitted leakage currents are different throughout the range of conditions in which they can be measured and the two values quoted are only examples.

Whenever new equipment is received into a hospital it should be subjected to an acceptance test which will verify that leakage currents and other characteristics affecting electrical safety are within the allowed specifications. Equipment should also be serviced regularly to ensure that its electrical safety does not become impaired.

Cardiac Pacemakers

Special risks apply to patients with cardiac pacemakers. Two types of pacemaker are used. First, for temporary use over a few days, a special pacemaker catheter can be inserted through the subclavian or jugular vein into the right ventricle. X-ray control is desirable, and full resuscitation facilities must be available during the procedure. Pulses of electric current are then passed through the electrode; the potential required to produce pacing of the heart is adjusted to the minimum needed, usually under 4 V, the pulse duration being under 1 ms.

The second form of pacemaker is for longer-term use. A battery-powered pacemaker and its pacing lead are embedded in the patient's tissues. Instead of an endocardial pacing lead, electrodes may be embedded in the myocardium, but then cardiac surgery is needed with exposure of the heart. Modern pacemakers are normally designed to work in a demand mode. This means that the stimulating electrode has a second function: it senses the electrical complexes from the atria and ventricles. The pacemaker then paces the heart only if the patient's heart rate is outside an acceptable range.

A problem with demand-mode pacemakers is that electromagnetic fields from sources outside the patient can cause interference (Fig. 16.7). The electrode of the pacemaker can act as an aerial and pick up signals from outside, then misinterpret them as QRS complexes. There are numerous possible sources of such interference: for example, electric motors, microwave ovens, and the antitheft devices found in shops and libraries. In the operating theatre, electrosurgical equipment, nerve stimulators and some monitoring equipment may carry risks. Magnetic resonance imaging (MRI) equipment and physiotherapy equipment can also interfere with the correct function of the pacemaker.

Figure 16.7 Interference at a demand-mode pacemaker from an external electromagnetic field

Source of interference

Pacemaker

Patients may experience dizziness and syncope when interference of this sort is present. Even the potentials from adjacent chest muscles can be picked up by the pacemaker and inhibit it. Many demand-mode pacemakers have an in-built safety factor in that they change to a fixed-rate mode when excessive interference is present. In addition, bipolar electrodes are available which have a connection to the atrium and ventricle and give more reliable detection of the ECG signal.

Conducting Fluids

Most of the infusion and other solutions used in hospitals are good conductors of electricity. These solutions are often used with or near to medical electrical equipment (e.g. infusion pumps), and great care should be taken to ensure that fluid is neither splashed nor allowed to enter equipment. If conducting solutions enter equipment, they may cause serious malfunction, and can be hydrolysed into an explosive mixture of hydrogen and oxygen by the passage of an electric current.

Power Failure

Failure of the mains electricity supply is another risk to patients, especially those on monitoring and life-support systems in theatre and intensive care areas. Most hospitals have provision for automatic connection of power supplies to an emergency generator, should mains failure occur. This risk is minimized further with some monitoring equipment which is battery operated and with ventilators which are powered from gas cylinders or a piped supply.

Equipment Containing Microprocessors

Much medical equipment contains microprocessors, which are essentially integrated electronic circuits performing data storage, computing and control functions. An example of their application is to be found in many infusion pumps, where infusion rates are set by pressing appropriate buttons; the entered values are then stored internally in electronic memory and used to control the infusion rate of the pump. There is a possibility that severe electrical interference may alter the stored values and, in the case of the infusion pump described, cause the pump to infuse at a different rate from that which was set by the user. Good circuit design can, however, provide a very large measure of protection against such faults.

Blood Pressure Measurement

Pressure at the Heart

Blood pressure arises from the force of contraction of the myocardium acting on the blood contained in the heart. The simple concept of pressure as force per unit area is less clear in this case because the force of contraction of the muscle is acting tangentially at the heart surface. This force gives rise to tension; in this context, tension is the force per unit length and Laplace's law (Chapter 2) applies.

Figure 17.1 shows a simple model of a spherical ventricle of a heart with a radius R. The pressure P resulting from tension T in the ventricular wall is determined by Laplace's law for a sphere as follows:

$$P = \frac{2T}{R}$$

The practical consequence of Laplace's law is that as a distended failing heart has a larger radius than normal, the distended myocardium is at a disadvantage in that the pressure produced falls unless the muscle contracts proportionately more forcefully. In the normal heart, however, slight distension caused by an increased venous return and the consequent lengthening of cardiac muscle increases the force of contraction (Starling's law of the heart) and the pressure is maintained.

The mechanical work of the heart for a single beat is related to the product of the pressure and the stroke volume (Chapter 8). Consequently, an increase of blood pressure or of stroke volume increases the work of the heart. Just as the elastic tissue in the lung stores the work of inspiration to power expiration, so the elastic tissue in the aorta and main vessels stores the work of the heart in systole to maintain blood flow during diastole.

Pressure in the Circulation

Blood pressure is not constant but varies with the site of measurement. Because the circulation is a system of tubes filled with a liquid, hydrostatic effects are present (Fig. 17.2).

In a tall man who is standing, the mean blood pressure could vary from 53 mmHg (7 kPa) at his head to 202 mmHg (27 kPa) at his feet, compared with a mean pressure of 90 mmHg (12 kPa) at his heart. This can be appreciated from Fig. 17.2, if it is remembered that 7.5 mmHg (1 kPa) equals 10 cmH$_2$O pressure. As blood pressure varies with site, a standard reference point is needed and this is generally accepted as being that of the level of the right atrium. The blood pressure also depends on the calibre of the vessel and its distance from the heart. Because there is a fall in pressure as a fluid flows through a tube, it might be expected that the mean pressure in arterioles would be lower than in arteries. This simple concept is complicated, however, by the fact that blood pressure is pulsatile

Figure 17.1 Application of Laplace's law to the heart

Figure 17.2 Hydrostatic effects on mean blood pressure

and changes in the wave pattern in different vessels alter the systolic pressures in them, as described later. In addition to changes in pressure depending on posture and site of measurement, blood pressure also shows a diurnal variation, being lower during sleep. Minor changes of pressure occur too during the respiratory cycle and more marked changes during intermittent positive pressure ventilation (IPPV), when, in addition to cyclical changes, there may be a general reduction in blood pressure due to the effects on venous return. Anxiety raises the blood pressure, so readings on three separate occasions may be required to obtain a representative value.

The total flow in the circulation, or the cardiac output, depends on the peripheral resistance and, if laminar flow is assumed,

$$\text{Peripheral resistance} = \frac{\text{Mean (aortic) blood pressure}}{\text{Cardiac output}}$$

Therefore:

Mean blood pressure = Peripheral resistance × Cardiac output

Thus, in a patient with a normal or low peripheral resistance (e.g. with a warm, pink skin) a high blood pressure indicates that a high cardiac output is likely, whereas a high blood pressure in a patient with a high peripheral resistance (e.g. with a cold, pale skin) may not indicate a raised cardiac output. In the formula the mean blood pressure is used. To obtain a fully accurate mean pressure, an integration technique would need to be applied to an arterial pressure trace. However, in practice, mean pressure can be estimated as diastolic pressure plus one-third of pulse pressure.

Measurement of Blood Pressure

The simplest noninvasive system of blood pressure measurement consists of an inflatable cuff connected to a manometer. The cuff is placed on the upper arm and the pressure at which the pulse returns after occlusion is identified by a detector system (Fig. 17.3).

Cuff

The cuff must be positioned so that the centre of its bladder is on the medial side of the arm over the brachial artery. The width of the cuff should be 20% greater than the diameter of the arm, d. The cuff with its tubing and connections should not leak.

Manometer

The mercury type of manometer must read zero correctly before use, and it should be used vertically unless it is of the type calibrated to be used at an angle. Partial blockage of the air vent or of the connecting tubings may lead to inaccurate or sluggish readings. Although aneroid gauges are more portable, their calibration should be checked regularly.

Detector

The cuff is inflated to a pressure above the expected systolic pressure, and this is then slowly released at a rate of 2–3 mmHg per second. The systolic pressure is indicated by the reappearance of the peripheral pulse, which can be monitored by a detector, the simplest form of which is manual palpation of the radial pulse. Auscultation over the brachial artery at the elbow allows detection of this point by the first-phase Korotkoff sound, i.e. the point at which sounds from blood flow in the artery first appear. The second phase is a slight muffling and the third phase is a rise in volume of the auscultation sounds. The fourth phase of Korotkoff sound is an abrupt fall in sound level and is sometimes taken as representing diastolic

Figure 17.3 Noninvasive measurement of blood pressure

Air vent

d

$d + 20\%$

Pulse detector

pressure, although the final loss of all sound (fifth phase of Korotkoff) is more widely accepted as indicating diastolic pressure.

A microphone with appropriate electronic circuitry is sometimes used in place of a stethoscope, particularly in apparatus intended for use by nonmedical or paramedical staff.

In anaesthesia, a pulse detector or pulse oximeter detector is often used on the patient's finger. This may then be used in conjunction with the standard blood pressure cuff, though the apparent systolic pressure indicated may be lower than the true systolic pressure.

Other more specialized detector systems are available and the oscillometric system, microphone detector or ultrasonic detector is particularly suited to the automated systems considered later.

Oscillometry

As the blood pressure cuff is deflated from a pressure above systolic pressure, the needle on an aneroid gauge will start to oscillate when systolic pressure is reached and this was used in one of the earliest techniques of blood pressure measurement. The oscillations of the needle increase in amplitude to a maximum at the mean blood pressure, then decrease at a less precise point about the diastolic pressure.

The Von Recklinghausen oscillotonometer improved on simple observation of the needle of an aneroid gauge, but electronic oscillometric equipment has now proved to be more convenient and accurate than the oscillotonometer and has the added advantage that it can provide automated measurement.

Automated Oscillometric Technique

Figure 17.4 illustrates the principles of the automated technique; instruments using this technique are known as noninvasive blood pressure (NIBP) monitors. Unlike the oscillotonometer, a single cuff is normally used and a pressure transducer measures both the pressure and the oscillations. The processing unit analyses the signal from the transducer to detect the onset of oscillations at the systolic pressure and the point of maximum oscillation at mean pressure, and to give an indi-

Figure 17.4 Principle of automatic blood pressure measurement

cation of the diastolic pressure. These can then be displayed. Most electronic oscil-lometric equipment has provision for automatic inflation of the cuff at preset inter-vals to a suitably high initial value, e.g. 160 mmHg, or, in repeated readings to 25 mmHg above the previous systolic measurement. During a reading, the pres-sure is slowly released by the bleed valve at 2–3 mmHg per second.

The frequency of cuff inflation is limited by the time required for the meas-urement process, and, apart from a mode in which measurements can be made repeatedly for a short period of time, most automated systems limit the rate at which readings can be made. If the interval between readings is too short, impeded blood flow may result, which is both clinically undesirable and liable to produce inaccurate results. A minimum interval of 2 min is preferable, except for short-term monitoring. The system gives reliable readings in adults and children pro-vided the appropriate cuff size is used, but, in common with other noninvasive techniques, results are less accurate if the patient has a dysrhythmia; also the appa-ratus fails to record at low pressures, e.g. below 50 mmHg.

Radial Artery Compression

To reduce the potential for injury resulting from repeated rapid inflation of a blood pressure cuff that occludes the circulation, an alternative technique uses a pressure sensor strapped to the wrist over the radial artery. The sensor is driven hydraulically by a control system to which it is attached and is used both to apply pressure to the wall of the radial artery and to measure pressure fluctuations at the wall of the artery due to pulsations during the cardiac cycle. As pressure is steadily increased from zero at the sensor, compressing the radial artery above the radius bone, the pressure fluctuations increase and then decrease, in a similar manner to the pulsations observed in the automated oscillometric technique. An algorithm in the control system determines the smallest sensor pressure at which the pressure oscillations are at their maximum value; this is the point at which maximum energy is transferred between the radial artery pulsations and the sensor. The algo-rithm then analyses pulsations near to this position and refers to a table of prede-termined values based on clinical data to derive systolic, diastolic and mean blood pressures. The system is also capable of displaying the shape of the blood pressure waveform. The technique is sensitive to motion artefact, but the algorithm con-tains a routine to detect motion and reject the measurement if this is identified.

Approximately 12–15 heart beats are required to obtain a measurement, so the system can provide more frequent measurements of blood pressure over a longer period than the automated oscillometric technique. Careful placement of the sensor is important to achieve good results.

The Penaz Technique

Figure 17.5 illustrates the principle of the Penaz technique, which is used to give continuous measurement of finger blood pressure. A cuff is placed on the finger attached to a transducer to measure pressure and to an air pump with a servo-control valve, as illustrated. In this respect, the technique resembles the electronic oscillometric technique and in its initial calibration, the apparatus detects the mean pressure from the point of maximum oscillation.

Unlike the oscillometric technique, the system also includes at the cuff an infrared light-emitting diode and a photocell which act as a photoplethysmograph. The photocell measures absorption at an infrared wavelength appropriate for

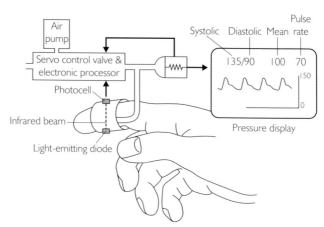

Figure 17.5 Penaz technique for the continuous measurement of blood pressure

arterial blood and so detects the volume of arterial blood in the finger under the cuff. The volume varies according to the degree of distension of the arteries during systole. An electronic processor analyses the photoplethysmograph to determine the volume at a point set according to the mean arterial pressure. Then the servocontrol valve at the air pump acts as a feedback mechanism, continuously inflating or deflating the finger cuff in order to maintain the photoplethysmograph output constant at this set point. The pressure at the transducer consequently gives a continuous tracing of arterial pressure. Some perfusion of the finger continues despite the continuous inflation of the finger cuff, but it remains to be seen if this perfusion is always adequate in long operations.

Other Automated Techniques

Alternatives to analysis of cuff pressure oscillations are possible. For example, a microphone may be positioned over the brachial artery to detect either audible sound or infrasound, i.e. low-frequency vibrations. Another technique which has been used incorporated an ultrasonic transmitter and receiver which were positioned, with appropriate gel for good transmission of sound, to detect the Doppler changes of frequency from arterial wall movement. A problem with both these systems is that it may be difficult to position the detectors correctly over the artery, in contrast to the oscillometric technique, which is less dependent on position.

All these techniques of automated blood pressure measurement give problems in patients with an irregular pulse, as pressure will vary from beat to beat. Also, the 1- or 2-min delay between readings may be unsatisfactory during operations when sudden changes of pressure are anticipated. Invasive techniques of blood pressure measurement therefore remain standard for patients in whom rapid changes of blood pressure are likely. Such situations occur, for example, following sudden blood loss, during operations for phaeochromocytoma or during controlled hypotension.

Invasive Techniques

If an artery is cannulated, a direct measurement of blood pressure can be obtained with the help of an infusion system, transducer and recorder.

Ideally, for arterial cannulation, a peripheral artery should be chosen so that the whole limb is not threatened if a clot or haematoma forms. Although some physicians use the brachial artery, the radial artery is usually the first choice but, before cannulation, a modified Allen test is carried out. The patient's hand is clenched into a fist and the doctor occludes both the radial and ulnar arteries with the fingers. Then the patient relaxes the clenched fist and the doctor releases the pressure on the ulnar artery. The patient's hand should then flush within 5 seconds. If flushing does not occur or is delayed, this indicates that there are poor blood vessel collaterals between the radial and ulnar arteries, and therefore another artery should be used. If the ulnar artery is to be cannulated the test is performed similarly, but pressure is released over the radial artery first.

If there are adequate connections between the two arteries, a plastic cannula may be inserted into the radial artery. A local anaesthetic is required in the conscious patient and the percutaneous route is usually satisfactory, open exposure rarely being necessary. Intra-arterial cannulation may rarely cause thrombosis to occur and to minimize this risk, the cannula should be constructed of Teflon, be short with parallel sides and be able to be sutured in place to avoid being dislodged.

After insertion, the cannula and its connections must be fixed securely, using Luer lock connections, so that there is no possibility of a leak occurring with the risk of severe or even fatal blood loss. To prevent clotting in the cannula, intermittent flushing with heparinized saline through a three-way tap may be satisfactory. However, the high pressures generated by small syringes (Chapter 1, Fig. 1.1) can damage arterial walls or the diaphragm of the pressure transducer. Care should be taken when catheters are being flushed, and syringes smaller than 5 ml should not be used. For longer-term recording, a continuous flushing system, as shown in Fig. 17.6, is more satisfactory.

The heparinized saline used is kept in a pressurized container at a pressure above systolic pressure. It then passes from the container through a constriction, adjusted so the flow cannot exceed about 4 ml per hour. This flow continuously flushes the tubing and the arterial cannula. Figure 17.6 also shows the pressure transducer with its amplifier and recorder, and such transducers are considered in Chapter 14.

Figure 17.6 Continuous flushing system for arterial pressure recording

Heparinized saline
300 mmHg (40 kPa)

Transducer

Amplifier

Constriction
4 ml per hour

Tap

Figure 17.7 Catheter tip transducer

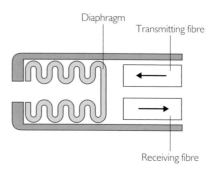

Fibreoptic Catheter Tip Transducer

The fibreoptic transducer-tipped pressure-monitoring catheter illustrated in Fig. 17.7 employs a mirror-coated moving diaphragm which reflects light carried to the tip by an optical fibre. The position of the diaphragm, which changes in response to changes in pressure, determines the fraction of the incident light that is reflected back down a second fibre. The other end of the catheter connects to an optoelectronic module which converts the light into an electrical signal. Associated electronics interpret the reflected light intensity in terms of pressure.

The Arterial Pressure Recording

The final waveform produced may be displayed on an oscilloscope or a recorder tracing. Figure 17.8 shows typical arterial pressure recordings. It can be seen that the form of the pressure wave alters as blood flows to the periphery. The blood pressure wave becomes narrower and increases in amplitude in peripheral arteries so that, even with the patient supine, the systolic pressure in the dorsalis pedis artery is higher than in the radial artery, which, in turn, is higher than that in the aorta. This modification of the wave pattern is caused by the change in diameter of the vessels and their elasticity, and possibly also because of the reflection of the wave pattern from the vessel walls.

The systolic and diastolic pressures are easily identified on a tracing and the systolic pressure is found to be an average of 5 mmHg higher with direct measurement at the radial artery than with indirect techniques, whereas the diastolic pressure is about 8 mmHg lower. The recording also shows the dicrotic notch caused by closure of the aortic valve.

Figure 17.8 Arterial pressure tracings from the aorta, the radial artery and the dorsalis pedis artery

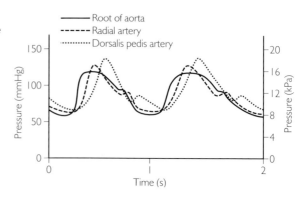

The frequency range of various biological signals is considered in Chapters 13 and 15. In the case of the arterial pressure wave, the frequency range is 0 Hz to about 40 Hz. The apparatus used for arterial pressure measurement must be able to respond adequately to this range of frequencies. Usually, the amplifiers and recorders have no difficulty in dealing with this frequency range, but problems may arise in relation to the transducer itself and its connections to the cannula.

Resonance and Damping

Movement of the diaphragm of the pressure transducer converts the blood pressure change into an electrical signal. This movement of the diaphragm is associated with a very small movement of saline to and fro along the catheter with changes of pressure. Just as a weight on the end of a spring will oscillate at a particular frequency (known as the resonant frequency), so the pressure-measuring system consisting of the transducer diaphragm, catheter and saline column possesses a resonant frequency at which oscillations can occur. If this is less than 40 Hz, it falls within the range of frequencies present in the blood pressure waveform. Oscillations occurring at the resonant frequency produce a sine wave which is superimposed on the blood pressure waveform, giving distortion from resonance, as shown in Fig. 17.9.

This problem can be avoided if the resonant frequency is outside the range of frequencies present in the blood pressure waveform, although this can be difficult to achieve. The resonant frequency of the combination of catheter and transducer can be raised most easily by using a shorter, wider or stiffer catheter, so the problem is generally worse when a long catheter is used.

If there is any restriction to the transmission of the blood pressure from the artery to the transducer diaphragm, the displayed blood pressure waveform will be damped or smoothed out so that sharp changes are not displayed (see Fig. 17.9). Damping of this sort can be produced by air bubbles in the catheter or in the transducer chamber, which absorb the pressure change in the saline column. It is also caused by clot formation in the cannula which restricts the movement of the saline column. Both these effects reduce the deflection of the transducer diaphragm, and hence the size of the measured waveform. Although resonance

Figure 17.9 Effect of resonance and damping on an arterial pressure trace

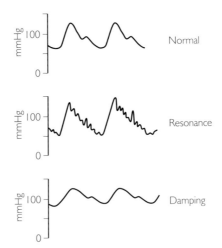

and damping can alter the measured values of systolic and diastolic pressure, the effect on the measured mean pressure is less.

Comparison of Invasive and Noninvasive Techniques

The main advantage of the direct invasive technique of arterial pressure measurement is its potential accuracy and its continuous display that permits an immediate response should a problem arise. It not only gives greater accuracy by indicating the exact form of the blood pressure trace but it can also give reliable pressure readings even in the most hypotensive or shocked patient, whereas noninvasive indirect techniques usually fail to record blood pressure below a certain minimum. The invasive method gives a continuous record of the pressure in contrast to the intermittent record provided by most noninvasive systems. Hence, it also gives better reliability than the noninvasive techniques if the pressure is continuously varying as, for example, in patients with an irregular or fluctuating pulse rate.

There are, however, disadvantages to the direct technique. There is some risk of arterial damage, whereas the noninvasive methods are harmless to the patient provided that measurements are not made too frequently. Direct systems are also more costly than the simpler indirect systems and there is a need for technical skill when using direct methods, whereas indirect techniques may be carried out by paramedical and even nonmedical staff.

Central Venous Pressure

The term blood pressure is normally used to refer to arterial blood pressure. However, the venous pressure is also of importance to anaesthetists. Accurate noninvasive measurement of this is impossible, although distended jugular veins in the absence of thoracic inlet obstruction indicate a raised venous pressure.

To measure central venous pressure, a catheter is inserted via an arm or neck vein and advanced so that it reaches the superior vena cava. Attached to this catheter are a saline drip, T-piece and a manometer, as shown in Fig. 17.10. The techniques used are beyond the scope of this book, but it should be noted that faulty techniques can increase the risk of pneumothorax, haemothorax or hydrothorax and of infection.

Before a central venous pressure reading is taken from the manometer, the patient is placed in a horizontal position. Using a spirit level on a rod attached to the manometer, the zero of the scale is set to the level of the midaxillary line, which is taken as representative of the level of the right atrium. The saline drip should be

Figure 17.10 Central venous pressure measurement

Midaxillary line

turned off when readings are made and slight movements of the saline level with respiration indicate correct positioning of the catheter. Readings are usually recorded as cmH_2O pressure, but conversion to SI units is simple as 1 cmH_2O is about 100 Pa. As an alternative to a simple saline manometer, a pressure transducer may be used and this also gives a continuous recording and allows identification of the central venous pressure waveform.

Venous Pressure and Cardiac Output

The filling of the heart depends on adequate venous pressure. If venous pressure rises, the normal heart fills to a greater extent and automatically increases its output even in the absence of autonomic innervation. The action is described by Starling's law of the heart, as described at the beginning of this chapter.

After appreciable blood loss, venous pressure falls and may be used as a guide to transfusion, but care is needed in interpreting venous pressure values as they can be modified by venous tone.

As shown in Fig. 17.11, both the right heart and pulmonary blood vessels are interposed between the central venous pressure recording point and the left heart.

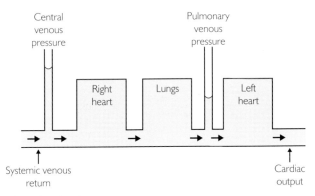

Figure 17.11 Central and pulmonary venous pressures

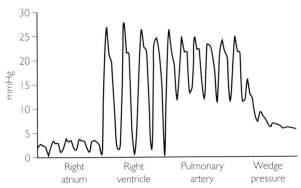

Figure 17.12 Pressure waveforms as a pulmonary artery catheter is advanced through the right heart and wedged in a pulmonary artery

Consequently, in a patient with left heart disease excessive intravenous transfusion can give pulmonary oedema before the warning sign of a high central venous pressure is seen. On the other hand, in a patient with lung disease, a high central venous pressure may be caused by failure of the right heart. Ideally, both left atrial and central venous pressures should therefore be monitored.

Measurement of pulmonary wedge pressure (Fig. 17.12) gives an indication of left atrial pressure. The pulmonary wedge pressure is obtained by advancing a special venous catheter through the right heart and pulmonary artery until it wedges into a small branch of the pulmonary artery, where it may be used to measure the pressure in the pulmonary capillaries. The special catheter used has a small balloon at its tip which can be inflated temporarily to facilitate its carriage into the pulmonary artery by the bloodstream. It is also inflated during wedge pressure measurement. Continuous pressure recording helps to identify the position of the catheter and ensure that it is positioned in the pulmonary vessels before making the measurement.

Oxygen Measurement

18

Clinical Assessment

Special techniques are required to measure the amount of oxygen in a patient's blood and respiratory gases, because clinical observation of the patient gives only limited information about oxygenation. For example, although hypoxia can stimulate tachypnoea via the carotid body receptors, this reflex is very variable and can be depressed by anaesthetics and other factors. Furthermore, there are many other possible causes of tachypnoea and it is thus an unreliable indication of hypoxia.

Another indirect indication of hypoxia in the patient is cyanosis. This too has limitations, as different observers may give different assessments of cyanosis and ambient lighting can bias judgement. It is particularly dangerous to assume that the absence of cyanosis indicates adequate oxygenation, because an anaemic patient may have a critically low oxygen saturation and yet not have sufficient deoxyhaemoglobin in the arterial blood to reveal cyanosis. (The term deoxyhaemoglobin is used in this chapter to indicate haemoglobin not combined with oxygen.)

Cyanosis indicates the presence of abnormally high concentrations of deoxyhaemoglobin in the blood in the capillaries, e.g. 50 g litre^{-1} or more. Cyanosis of the lips can normally be assumed to indicate reduced oxygen saturation in the arterial blood. However, in patients with a reduced cardiac output or in capillaries where stasis is present, cyanosis may be unrelated to arterial saturation.

These problems in the clinical assessment of cyanosis are avoided if a sample of arterial blood is taken anaerobically, heparinized and examined in suitable apparatus. If an even more complete assessment of hypoxia in the patient is needed then, in addition, a mixed venous sample may be taken from a central venous catheter.

Spectrophotometric Measurements of Oxygen Saturation

Spectrophotometric techniques of measurement involve passing radiation through a sample and determining the quantity of radiation absorbed. The wavelength of the radiation is chosen so that it is absorbed by the compound of interest in the sample. There are two laws which describe how radiation is absorbed as it passes through a sample or a solution:

Beer's law states that the absorption of radiation by a given thickness of a solution of a given concentration is the same as that of twice the thickness of a solution of half the concentration.

Bouguer's or Lambert's law states that each layer of equal thickness absorbs an equal fraction of radiation which passes through it.

These laws may be combined to describe the absorption of radiation by a sample in general. The absorption of radiation by the compound of interest in a sample increases as the concentration increases. At sufficiently low concentrations, the absorption is proportional to the concentration.

A spectrophotometric technique may be used to assess the amount of deoxyhaemoglobin in the blood in an instrument known as an oximeter. In an oximeter, light of various wavelengths is transmitted through a haemolysed blood sample and a photocell detects the light absorbances so that the oxygen saturation can be calculated.

Figure 18.1 illustrates the physical principle underlying the working of the instrument. The light absorbed by blood depends on the quantities of deoxyhaemoglobin and oxyhaemoglobin present and the wavelength of the light. As shown in the figure the absorbance of oxyhaemoglobin in red light at a wavelength of 660 nm is less than that of deoxyhaemoglobin and this accounts for its red appearance. In the infrared region, e.g. at 940 nm, the absorbance of deoxyhaemoglobin is less than that of oxyhaemoglobin. Comparison of the absorbances at these wavelengths enables an oximeter to calculate the oxygen saturation. The points at which the absorbances for the two forms of haemoglobin are identical are known as 'isobestic points' and the absorbance at any of these points depends only on the haemoglobin concentration. Earlier models of an oximeter used a wavelength at an isobestic point to compensate for haemoglobin concentration but current oximeters use various wavelengths to derive the results and give a direct reading of saturation and, if needed, total haemoglobin content.

Figure 18.2 gives a simplified illustration of an oximeter. The blood sample to be analysed is drawn up into the apparatus by a system of pumps to be diluted and haemolysed before entering the cuvette. Light passes through filter A to provide a monochromatic beam – i.e. of a single wavelength – and this light passes through the cuvette of haemolysed blood and is then detected by a photocell shown on the right. A second photocell acts as a reference detector, picking up a fixed fraction of the light deflected by the beam splitter as shown, so that a comparison of the output of the two detectors allows computation of the oxygen saturation of the blood and of the total haemoglobin, if required. Figure 18.2 shows one lamp

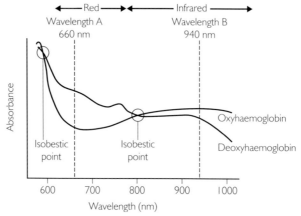

Figure 18.1 Variation of the absorption of light according to its wavelength by oxyhaemoglobin and deoxyhaemoglobin

Figure 18.2 Principle of the oximeter

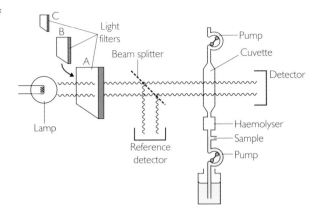

and filters which could be mounted on a rotating disc, but oximeters may instead use several light-emitting diodes, designed to give light at appropriate wavelengths, which can be switched on and off in rapid sequence.

Correction for Carboxyhaemoglobin

The effects of traces of carbon monoxide in the blood may be important, especially in cigarette smokers, in whom up to 15% of haemoglobin can be in the form of carboxyhaemoglobin due to inhaled carbon monoxide. City dwellers may also have small amounts of carboxyhaemoglobin in their blood from carbon monoxide in the air.

The oximeter illustrated avoids errors from the presence of carboxyhaemoglobin by careful selection of the light wavelengths used in analysis and by electronic computation. In addition, carboxyhaemoglobin may be measured by using a series of light filters or diodes for differing frequencies of light. Oximeters are now available using a range of wavelengths to measure other forms of haemoglobin, including methaemoglobin.

In addition to its use in oximeters that analyse haemolysed blood *in vitro*, the principle described above is used in the pulse oximeter for the measurement of oxygen saturation *in vivo*.

Pulse Oximeter

Figure 18.3 illustrates the principle of the pulse oximeter. Radiation from red (660 nm) and infrared (940 nm) light-emitting diodes passes through a finger and the photocell shown detects the transmitted radiation. The output of the sensor is processed electronically to give a pulse waveform and the arterial oxygen saturation. Appropriate sensors are also available for use on the ear.

As in the previously described oximeters, the diodes are switched on and off in sequence, with a pause during which both diodes are off. This pause allows the photocell and microprocessor to detect and compensate for any ambient light which may have penetrated round the sensor cover. The diodes are switched on and off at high frequency, several hundred times a second. Consequently, this does not prevent the oximeter detecting the cyclical changes in the signal caused by arterial pulsations during the cardiac cycle. A microprocessor is programmed to

Figure 18.3 Principle of the pulse oximeter

analyse these changes of light absorption during the arterial pulsatile flow and ignore the nonpulsatile component of the signal due to the tissues and venous blood. The pulse oximeter can thus give a satisfactory reading of arterial oxygen saturation.

Pulse oximeters which use only two diodes do not compensate fully for carboxyhaemoglobin or other abnormal haemoglobins. Moreover, different models of pulse oximeter are not all equally accurate at low oxygen saturation or in cases of peripheral vasoconstriction and some pulse oximeters may be slow in their response to a fall in arterial oxygen saturation, particularly if a finger sensor rather than an ear sensor is used. Pigments on the fingernail or skin staining may also affect the results. Despite these limitations, the pulse oximeter is established as one of the most important monitors for routine use in anaesthesia.

A further problem to be overcome in the analysis of the signal waveforms generated by the sensor is rejection of movement artefact, which results in changes in the transmitted radiation that are not due to arterial pulsations. One technique is to average the results over a number of consecutive waveforms, so the effect of the movement artefact is reduced. An alternative technique makes the assumption that movements cause pulsation in the venous signal and that this signal has a lower oxygen saturation than the arterial signal. Signal processing identifies the two different values of oxygen saturation that are present, separates the venous and arterial signals and allows measurement of the arterial signal alone.

A device has been introduced for clinical use which permits monitoring of the cytochrome redox state in order to assess the degree of oxygenation in the brain. It is a noninvasive system which, like the pulse oximeter, uses absorption of light as a measuring technique but operates in the near infrared using a low-power semiconductor laser as a light source.

Oxygen Content

The measurement of oxyhaemoglobin gives an indication of the oxygen content of the blood, provided that the haemoglobin concentration and its oxygen combining power are known and that the oxygen in solution in the plasma is taken into account:

Oxygen content = (Blood oxygen saturation × Haemoglobin concentration × Oxygen combining power of haemoglobin) + Oxygen in solution

It is more accurate to measure the oxygen content of the blood sample directly. In one type of apparatus which has been used for this, oxygen is flushed out of a haemolysed blood sample by means of an oxygen-free carrier gas and the total oxygen content in the gas measured with a fuel cell.

Interrelation of Oxygen Saturation and Oxygen Tension

As an alternative to oxygen saturation measurement, the oxygen tension (PO_2) of blood can be measured and there is a relatively consistent relationship between these measurements, as shown by the oxygen dissociation curve (Fig. 18.4). Some instruments which measure PO_2 also compute the saturation automatically after compensating for the effects of blood hydrogen ion concentration (H^+) on the curve. This is not ideal because, in addition to (H^+), the curve is affected by other factors, including the level of 2,3-diphosphoglycerate (DPG) in the red blood cells, and direct measurement gives better accuracy than computation. Figure 18.4 also shows the value of P_{50}, which is the partial pressure of oxygen when 50% of the haemoglobin is saturated. The value of P_{50} reflects the left or right shift of the dissociation curve; the normal value is 3.58 kPa (26.8 mmHg). A typical value for venous oxygen saturation, 74%, is also shown, which corresponds to a PO_2 of 5.33 kPa (40 mmHg).

At lower than normal oxygen saturation, a small change of PO_2 is associated with a large change in saturation; hence, oxygen saturation measurement may give a more accurate indication of a patient's oxygenation. In addition, of the two measurements, oxygen saturation is normally more relevant to patient care because it gives an index of the oxygen content of the blood and so of the oxygen which can be supplied to the tissues. Although PO_2 gives a measure of the partial pressure available for diffusion of the oxygen across membranes and capillaries, this is probably less important because oxygen diffuses readily across the pulmonary capillaries (Chapter 7), and because the mitochondria in the tissues can still use oxygen at tensions of a small fraction of a kilopascal (i.e. a few mmHg).

In respiratory study measurements, however, it is often necessary to measure high values of saturation or tension, and in this range a large change of PO_2 is associated with a range of 98–100% in saturation, so PO_2 measurement gives greater sensitivity.

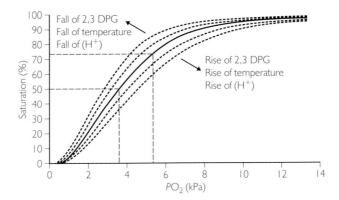

Figure 18.4 Oxygen dissociation curve

Measurement of Oxygen Tension

Blood gas analysers are available which allow measurement of the oxygen tension in a sample of blood in addition to measurement of the carbon dioxide tension and the pH of the sample. For oxygen tension measurements, the apparatus incorporates an oxygen electrode, also known as a Clark electrode or a polarographic electrode. The principle of this electrode is illustrated in Fig. 18.5.

A platinum cathode and a silver/silver chloride anode are shown in a solution of electrolyte such as potassium chloride. A voltage of 0.6 V is applied between the electrodes, and the current flow is measured. At the anode, electrons are provided by the reaction of silver with the chloride ions of the potassium chloride electrolyte to give silver chloride and electrons. At the cathode, oxygen combines with the electrons and water, giving rise to hydroxyl ions:

$$O_2 + 4e + 2H_2O \rightarrow 4OH^-$$

The more oxygen available, the more electrons which can be taken up at the cathode and, consequently, the greater the current flow. So the current flow through the cell is dependent on the oxygen tension at the platinum cathode.

The reaction at the cathode is analogous to that occurring in cell mitochondria (Fig. 18.6). In this case, the electrons produced in the Krebs cycle are transmitted down the chain of respiratory enzymes. In this respiratory chain, oxygen combines with the electrons to give rise to hydroxyl ions, while at the same time adenosine triphosphate (ATP) is formed from adenosine diphosphate (ADP).

The platinum cathode of the oxygen electrode cannot be inserted directly into the blood because deposits of protein form and affect its function; thus, as shown in

Figure 18.5 Principle of the oxygen electrode

Figure 18.6 Krebs cycle and respiratory enzyme chain

Figure 18.7 Oxygen
electrode

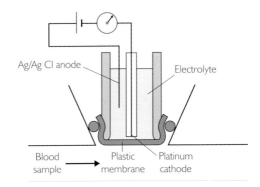

Ag/Ag Cl anode

Electrolyte

Blood
sample

Plastic
membrane

Platinum
cathode

Fig. 18.7, there is a plastic membrane separating the blood from a small amount of electrolyte lying over the tip of the platinum cathode. The oxygen tension in the blood equilibrates with that in the electrolyte around the cathode and the reaction described above takes place, so that the current flow is dependent on the oxygen tension at the cathode. Temperature control is important, so the electrode is maintained at 37°C during use. Standard gas mixtures are normally employed for electrode calibration.

The oxygen electrode must be kept scrupulously clean to prevent contamination, and its plastic membrane should be checked and replaced if punctured or if deposits of protein form on it. The arterial blood sample must be taken anaerobically and heparinized to prevent clotting, and analysis must be made promptly, as the oxygen tension in an arterial blood sample falls steadily, particularly if it is maintained at room temperature. This fall in oxygen concentration is caused by the metabolism in the cells in the blood. If delay is unavoidable, then a correction factor is sometimes applied to allow for the time since the sample was taken. Alternatively, samples may be placed in a receptacle full of ice to reduce the rate of fall of the oxygen tension. These techniques are less accurate, however, than immediate analysis of the sample.

A miniature oxygen electrode mounted on the tip of a catheter has been produced to allow continuous measurement of the oxygen tension of blood inside blood vessels and the heart. It readily shows changes in oxygen tension, but calibration is more difficult than with the conventional larger apparatus described.

As well as its use for measuring the tension of oxygen in blood samples, the polarographic oxygen electrode may also be used for measuring the concentration of oxygen in gas mixtures. In portable oxygen monitors using the polarographic electrode, the electrolyte is in the form of a gel, but this and the membrane deteriorate fairly rapidly with use and must be replaced.

False high readings may arise when some oxygen electrodes are used in the presence of halothane, as the anaesthetic is reduced by the polarizing voltage of 0.6 V. However, the use of an electrode membrane which is not readily permeable to halothane can minimize this problem.

The Fuel Cell

Although the oxygen electrode may be used to measure the partial pressure of oxygen in gas mixtures, in practice several other types of apparatus are commonly used for this purpose. The fuel cell is considered first as it has some similarities to the oxygen electrode.

Figure 18.8 illustrates the similarity between the oxygen electrode and the fuel cell. In the oxygen electrode there is a platinum cathode, whereas in the fuel cell the cathode is in the form of a gold mesh. However, the reactions at the cathode are the same in both cases:

$$O_2 + 4e + 2H_2O \rightarrow 4OH^-$$

The current flow depends on the uptake of oxygen at the cathode and thus on the partial pressure of oxygen. The anodes, however, are different in the two cases. In the oxygen electrode, there is a silver/silver chloride wire anode, but in the fuel cell the anode is made of lead and the electrolyte is potassium hydroxide. At the anode, electrons are produced by the combination of hydroxyl ions from the potassium hydroxide electrolyte with the lead as follows:

$$Pb + 2OH^- \rightarrow PbO + H_2O + 2e$$

Unlike the oxygen electrode, no battery is needed in the fuel cell because the cell produces a voltage, thus acting as a battery. Like other batteries it eventually expires, and the actual life of the cell depends on the period during which it is exposed to oxygen, which may be several months. As with the polarographic electrode, temperature affects the output of a fuel cell, but temperature compensation may be achieved by means of a thermistor placed within the fuel cell, as shown in Fig. 18.8.

The cell is connected to a small indicator unit to provide a portable and reliable oxygen analyser for clinical and bedside use. A typical cell has a response time of about 30 s. Although this type of analyser is not expensive, the detector cells have a limited life span and do need replacing. Additionally, if a standard cell is used in the presence of nitrous oxide, nitrous oxide diffuses into the cell. At the anode the nitrous oxide reacts with the lead in the presence of the electrolyte to produce nitrogen, which alters the pressure inside the cell and may damage it. Nevertheless, there are special cells designed for use in anaesthetic practice when nitrous oxide might be present, but they have a shorter life span than the standard ones.

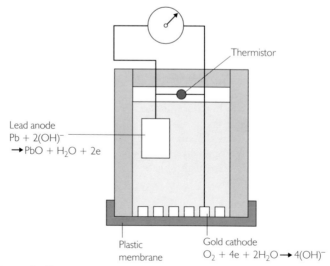

Figure 18.8 Fuel cell

Although the fuel cell oxygen sensor has a slower response than the polaro-graphic type, it requires less maintenance and has a guaranteed life span.

Paramagnetic Analyser

Another technique for measuring the concentration of oxygen in gases is based on the fact that oxygen is paramagnetic and is, therefore, attracted into a magnetic field (Fig. 18.9).

On the other hand, most other gases, e.g. nitrogen, are weakly diamagnetic and are repelled from a magnetic field. The paramagnetic property of oxygen arises from its molecular structure, being due to the fact that the electrons in the outer shell of an oxygen molecule are unpaired. In the paramagnetic oxygen analyser, a gas-tight chamber or cell containing two glass spheres connected in a dumb-bell arrangement is placed in a nonuniform magnetic field (Fig. 18.10).

The dumb-bell is suspended on a filament so that it can rotate, and the glass spheres are filled with nitrogen. The zero reading of the instrument may be adjusted by filling the chamber around the spheres with nitrogen. The orientation of the dumb-bell in the magnetic field is determined by the tension of the suspending fila-ment. Suppose oxygen is added to the cell; the oxygen is attracted into the magnetic field and tends to displace the glass spheres containing nitrogen. The dumb-bell therefore rotates until the force of this displacement is balanced by the tension of the filament. This deflection of the dumb-bell may be measured by attaching a mirror to

Figure 18.9 Paramagnetic property of oxygen

Figure 18.10 Simple paramagnetic oxygen analyser

the dumb-bell suspension as illustrated, so that the position of a light beam reflected from this mirror provides an indication on a scale. The scale can be calibrated to give the percentage of oxygen present in the measuring cell.

Figure 18.11 illustrates an alternative paramagnetic technique. The reflected light beam falls on two photocells, and the output from these is compared and used to generate a current that flows through a coil around the dumb-bell. This current produces an opposing magnetic field which keeps the dumb-bell in its resting position. The amount of current required to keep the dumb-bell steady gives a measure of the concentration of oxygen in the cell. Such null-deflection analysers give very accurate results, typically 0.1%.

The principle of a further type of paramagnetic oxygen analyser, which has the advantage of containing no moving parts, is shown in Fig. 18.12. A differential pressure transducer measures the difference in pressure between two streams of gas – a sample gas and a reference gas. The reference gas can be air. Both streams of gas flow through a region in which there is a pulsed magnetic field that is generated by an electromagnet, the current through which is switched on and off. When the magnetic field is switched on, oxygen molecules are attracted into the field. The movement of oxygen molecules into the magnetic field causes a reduction of pressure in the volume of gas situated between the magnetic field and the flow restriction upstream of the field. This reduction in pressure causes a deflection of the pressure transducer diaphragm towards the connection to the gas stream with the greater oxygen concentration, as illustrated in the figure by the dashed line in the differential pressure transducer. When the magnetic field is switched off, the differential pressure is no longer present and the transducer diaphragm returns to its

Figure 18.11 Null-deflection type of paramagnetic oxygen analyser

Figure 18.12 Pulsed-field paramagnetic oxygen analyser

central position. There is thus an alternating pressure at the transducer, the magnitude of which is a measure of the oxygen partial pressure in the sample gas.

Analysis of Gases Containing Water Vapour

Water vapour has the potential to affect the accuracy of many gas analysers. If water vapour is added to a previously dry mixture of gases, the concentration of the other components will be reduced because of the partial pressure of the water vapour. This may sometimes be important. Consider, for example, the measurement of the oxygen consumption of a patient who inspires dry gas but who expires humidified gas. Unless a correction is made for the addition of water vapour to the gas mixture, the oxygen consumption result will be inaccurate.

If humidified gases are analysed at 37°C, the oxygen concentration in the dry mixture can be calculated from the partial pressure of oxygen, the barometric pressure and the saturated vapour pressure (SVP) of water at 37°C:

$$\text{Concentration} = \frac{\text{Partial pressure (humidified at 37°C)}}{\text{Barometric pressure} - \text{SVP of water at 37°C}}$$

As an alternative to calculation, water vapour may be removed by passing the gases through a drying agent such as silica gel before analysis. Many gas analysers now contain special tubing which removes water vapour before the sample reaches the sample cell.

Continuous in-vivo Oxygen Measurement

Most of the instruments described are used for intermittent sampling of arterial blood, mixed venous blood or gas samples, but in the seriously ill patient, a single reading may not be representative and continuous recording of the oxygen tension may be desirable. Several techniques are available to meet this need. Thus, a miniaturized polarographic electrode may be used in a catheter in an artery, or in a central venous line. The mass spectrometer (Chapter 20) has been used to give a continuous measurement of oxygen tension using an intravascular catheter.

Unfortunately, calibration remains a problem with most of the continuous recording systems. Consequently, serial sampling from an indwelling arterial catheter or from a central venous line is still used in the management of the seriously ill patient. However, an alternative technique, that of transcutaneous oxygen measurement, is useful as a complement to blood gas analysis, particularly in neonates.

Transcutaneous Oxygen Measurement

At room temperature, some of the oxygen supplied by the peripheral circulation is used in metabolism by the tissues underlying the skin surface. However, if the skin is heated locally to 43–44°C, the peripheral blood vessels dilate and the oxygen used in the skin is negligible compared with the total oxygen present in the capillaries. The skin and capillary tensions then approximate to the arterial tension. Since oxygen diffuses through the skin, an oxygen electrode placed on the skin surface can be used to measure the arterial oxygen tension.

A cross section through a typical transcutaneous oxygen electrode is shown in Fig. 18.13. A platinum or gold cathode is surrounded by a silver anode, both electrodes being in contact with a thin layer of electrolyte retained by a membrane

Figure 18.13
Transcutaneous oxygen electrode

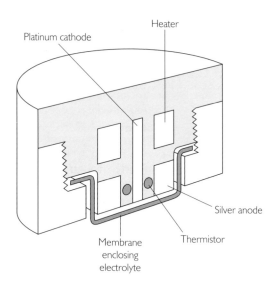

permeable to oxygen. The complete system forms a polarographic electrode, the operation of which has been described above. The skin temperature is measured by a thermistor, and this is used to control the heater power. Failure of the temperature control system is dangerous, as burns can occur if the skin temperature rises above 45°C (Chapter 9). Consequently, a second thermistor is used to switch off the heater if the primary heating circuit fails. Nevertheless, to avoid damage to the skin and to maintain accurate operation, the electrode position should be changed every 3–6 hours.

Transcutaneous oxygen measurement is less accurate than analysis of blood samples, but as it is continuous it can be used to complement the latter. Inaccuracies arise from the metabolism of oxygen as it diffuses through the skin, the shift in the oxygen dissociation curve with temperature, and the reduction of skin perfusion due to oedema resulting from the high operating temperature of the electrode. Inaccurate low readings also arise if cardiac output falls, as skin perfusion is then reduced. The response time of the transcutaneous electrode is rather slow. The electrode responds in about 1 min to changes of oxygen tension at its surface. Furthermore, the changes in cutaneous tension in turn lag behind changes in arterial blood tension.

Hydrogen Ion and Carbon Dioxide Measurement

19

Hydrogen Ion Concentration and pH

pH is a measure of the hydrogen ion activity in a liquid. Hydrogen ion activity is not exactly the same as hydrogen ion concentration [H⁺] but, for practical purposes in the clinical situation, these may be regarded as equivalent. The pH is defined as the negative logarithm to the base 10 of [H⁺]; hence, a [H⁺] of 10^{-9} mol litre^{-1} is a pH of 9. Each decrease of one pH unit is equivalent to a 10-fold increase of [H⁺]:

pH of 9 = 1 nmol litre^{-1} [H⁺] or 10^{-9} mol litre^{-1}

pH of 8 = 10 nmol litre^{-1} [H⁺] or 10^{-8} mol litre^{-1}

pH of 7 = 100 nmol litre^{-1} [H⁺] or 10^{-7} mol litre^{-1}

pH of 7.4 = 40 nmol litre^{-1} [H⁺] or $10^{-7.4}$ mol litre^{-1}

The normal blood [H⁺] is 40 nmol litre^{-1} at 37°C, and this is equal to a pH of 7.4. As illustrated on the graph (Fig. 19.1), the relationship between [H⁺] and pH is approximately linear over the middle of the clinical range, the pH decreasing by approximately 0.1 for each 10 nmol litre^{-1} increase in [H⁺]. Thus, 50 nmol litre^{-1} corresponds to a pH of 7.3. Details of the clinical problems surrounding the maintenance of the acid–base state of the blood are beyond the scope of this book.

Measurement of [H⁺]

Figure 19.2 illustrates a [H⁺] electrode assembly. The [H⁺] electrode is an example of an ion-selective electrode and it depends for its operation on the hydrogen ion sensitive glass shown at its tip. A potential develops across this glass which

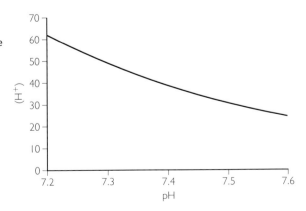

Figure 19.1 Relationship of [H⁺] in nmol litre^{-1} to pH over the middle of the clinical range

Figure 19.2 Hydrogen ion measurement system; most systems in clinical use also include PCO_2 and PO_2 electrodes

depends on the difference of [H⁺] across it. The [H⁺] within the [H⁺] electrode is maintained at a constant value by a buffer solution, so the potential across the glass is dependent on the [H⁺] in the blood sample in the channel illustrated. To measure the potential difference it is necessary to make electrical contact with the blood and with the buffer solution. In the case of the blood, a reference electrode is used which has a membrane at its tip to avoid contamination. In both the [H⁺] electrode and the reference electrode, stability of the metal to solution contact is achieved through a special electrode of silver in contact with its chloride, which is in contact in turn with a solution of chloride ions. The silver/silver chloride connection in the [H⁺] electrode is then in contact with the buffer solution shown while the silver/silver chloride connection of the reference electrode is linked to the membrane and blood via a saturated solution of potassium chloride which completes the electric circuit. The potential difference between the electrodes is measured and converted to a direct reading of [H⁺] or pH as required.

There is an automatic suction control to draw the blood through the channel. Automatic systems of this type are often arranged as part of a comprehensive electrode system which measures oxygen and carbon dioxide tensions in addition to [H⁺]. Normally, the blood sample is an arterial blood sample which is taken anaerobically and heparinized and analysed promptly.

Temperature control is important when measuring [H⁺]. Consequently, as seen in Fig. 19.2, the electrodes and the blood channel are surrounded by a thermal control system to maintain the temperature at 37°C. Dissociation of acids and bases increases with temperature and thus alterations in temperature change the [H⁺]. If the blood sample is not at 37°C – e.g. from a patient under hypothermic conditions – then a correction factor may be used to indicate the true [H⁺] in the patient.

Before use, the apparatus must be calibrated with two buffer solutions, each containing a fixed concentration of two phosphate buffers, for which the hydrogen ion concentration has been decided by international agreement. In addition, the electrode system must be carefully maintained to ensure accuracy. Any membrane must be clean and have no holes in it and electrodes must be regularly cleaned to remove any protein material which tends to accumulate on them.

In addition to the use of the apparatus for blood samples it may also be used for [H+] measurements in urine and in cerebrospinal fluid.

Ion-selective electrodes other than the [H+] electrode are available, their different properties being achieved with the use of appropriate glass in their construction. Thus it is possible to measure the concentration of an ion such as K^+, Na^+ or Ca^{2+} with an electrode which works on the same principle as the [H+] electrode, but is made of glass which responds specifically to one of these ions.

Measurement of PCO_2

The carbon dioxide tension in arterial blood ($PaCO_2$) is a valuable measurement of the adequacy of a patient's ventilation, the tension of carbon dioxide in blood being the partial pressure of carbon dioxide which would be in equilibrium with the blood. The normal $PaCO_2$ is 5.3 kPa or 40 mmHg.

The main methods of measuring the PCO_2 of liquids are based on [H+] measurement because carbon dioxide reacts with water to produce hydrogen ions by the reversible reactions:

$$CO_2 + H_2O \leftrightarrow H_2CO_3^- \leftrightarrow H^+ + HCO_3^-$$

The first reaction gives carbonic acid which, in turn, dissociates to produce hydrogen ions and bicarbonate ions. The carbon dioxide tension is therefore related to the hydrogen ion concentration. This interrelationship of PCO_2 is used in the Severinghaus CO_2 electrode.

Figure 19.3 illustrates the Severinghaus CO_2 electrode, which provides a direct method of PCO_2 measurement from the [H+] change. The apparatus incorporates hydrogen ion sensitive glass, shown in the centre, with electrodes either side of it. This glass is in contact with a thin film of sodium bicarbonate solution in a nylon mesh, which is fixed over the glass tip by means of an O-ring. The liquid to be tested, usually arterial blood, is separated from the nylon mesh and bicarbonate by a plastic membrane that is permeable to carbon dioxide and is also attached by means of an O-ring. At the tip of the electrode, carbon dioxide diffuses through the plastic membrane into the mesh impregnated with the bicarbonate solution and combines with the water present as described above. The resulting change of [H+] is measured by the glass electrode.

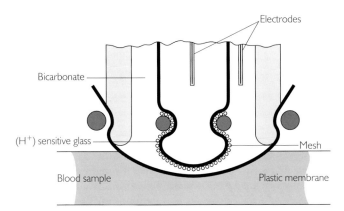

Figure 19.3 Severinghaus CO_2 electrode

If a small hole occurs in the plastic membrane, it ceases to be a semipermeable membrane for carbon dioxide and the apparatus becomes inaccurate, but with care an accuracy of about 130 Pa (1 mmHg) may be obtained. The response time of the electrode is about 2–3 min, being slower than the [H$^+$] electrode because the carbon dioxide requires time to diffuse through the plastic membrane. As with the [H$^+$] electrode, the carbon dioxide must be maintained at 37°C and calibrated before use with standard gas mixtures containing known concentrations of carbon dioxide. As the meter gives readings as tensions or partial pressures in kPa or mmHg, it is necessary to convert the concentrations of the calibration mixtures to partial pressures. It must be remembered that, although the partial pressure of a dry gas can be obtained by multiplying the concentration by the barometric pressure, for humidified gas the saturated vapour pressure of water must be subtracted from the barometric pressure.

In the blood gas apparatus, the calibration mixtures are fully humidified on their way to the electrode. An example of the calibration for carbon dioxide is as follows. If the barometric pressure is 100 kPa and the saturated vapour pressure of water at 37°C is 6.3 kPa, a 5% carbon dioxide concentration calibrating gas gives a partial pressure of 4.7 kPa:

$$\frac{5}{100} \times (100 - 6.3) \text{ kPa} = 4.7 \text{ kPa}$$

The calculation in terms of millimetres of mercury is

$$\frac{5}{100} \times (750 - 47) \text{ mmHg} = 35 \text{ mmHg}$$

For a 5% carbon dioxide calibrating gas in this example, therefore, the meter calibration must be set to read 4.7 kPa or 35 mmHg, depending on the machine.

The $PaCO_2$ provides a measure of the carbon dioxide in solution in the blood. However, this is only a small part of the total carbon dioxide, which also includes carbon dioxide combined as bicarbonate and carbonate and in association with haemoglobin. However, in anaesthesia the $PaCO_2$ is the most important measurement.

In the same way that transcutaneous oxygen electrodes can be used to measure oxygen tensions (Chapter 18), transcutaneous carbon dioxide electrodes are available which use a similar temperature control system but which use an electrode of the Severinghaus type.

Infrared Analyser

An instrument which gives a continuous recording of carbon dioxide concentration is known as a capnograph; the infrared analyser may be used for this purpose and for the measurement of the concentration of many other gases.

Gases that have two or more different atoms in the molecule absorb infrared radiation and by measuring the fraction of radiation absorbed by a gas mixture, the partial pressure of a particular gas can be determined. Each gas absorbs radiation at a characteristic wavelength. The proportion of radiation absorbed also depends on the wavelength, as shown in Fig. 19.4. By careful choice of an infrared wavelength and by taking into account the potential components of a gas mixture, it is possible to measure the gas of interest and avoid interference from other gases. As an example, Fig. 19.4 shows that the use of infrared radiation with a wavelength of 4.28 μm for the analysis of carbon dioxide should reduce interference from the presence of nitrous oxide.

Figure 19.4 Absorption of infrared radiation by carbon dioxide and nitrous oxide depends on the wavelength of the radiation

The principle of an infrared analyser is shown in Fig. 19.5. The infrared radiation is emitted by a hot wire and the particular frequency required is obtained by passing the radiation through a filter. An instrument designed to analyse the concentration of carbon dioxide alone could have a filter which passes one chosen wavelength, whereas more versatile instruments incorporate variable filters so radiation wavelengths appropriate to a variety of different gases may be selected. The principle resembles that described in the spectrophotometric analysis of oxygen saturation (Chapter 18) and, as in the oximeter, the filters can be mounted on a rotating disc to permit simultaneous analysis of several sample compounds. The rotating disc or chopper has the added advantage that it causes an alternating signal to fall on the detector. This is easier to amplify and is less prone to drift than a steady signal. As glass absorbs infrared radiation, the sample chamber has windows made from a material which is transparent to infrared radiation, such as sapphire.

After passing through the sample chamber the radiation is focused on a photodetector. The greater the absorption of infrared radiation by the gas being measured in the sample, the less the radiation monitored by the detector. Consequently it is possible to process the detector output electronically to indicate the concentration of gas present.

Figure 19.5 Infrared analyser

Variations in the output of the detector may also be caused by changes in the output of the infrared source and the sensitivity of the detector, and variation in transmission of the optical components in the system. To avoid such variations being interpreted as changes in the concentration of carbon dioxide in the sample cell, some instruments use a second beam of radiation from the same source which passes through a reference cell containing carbon dioxide free air. Changes of output which are not due to changes of carbon dioxide concentration in the sample cell also appear at a reference detector and may be subtracted from the output of the sample detector. An analyser of this type is known as a double beam instrument.

Various physical processes result in gas molecules absorbing radiation over a restricted range of wavelengths centred about a peak, as shown in Fig. 19.4, rather than at a specific single wavelength. One of these processes is due to intermolecular forces, which vary as the distance between individual molecules varies. As the molecules approach and recede from each other, their energies alter slightly and this affects the energy at which they absorb infrared radiation. The effect is known as the collision broadening effect. The interaction between different types of molecules is generally different from the interaction between the same type of molecule, so if nitrous oxide is added to a gas mixture, the wavelengths at which the absorption of infrared radiation by carbon dioxide molecules takes place is affected. As most anaesthetic mixtures contain nitrous oxide, most analysers provide compensation for its presence, either as a manual adjustment in which the anaesthetist keys in the percentage in use, or automatic compensation in which the analyser uses the percentage of nitrous oxide obtained from infrared analysis of the mixture.

Figure 19.6 shows the two types of capnograph – the side-stream and main-stream capnographs. In the side-stream capnograph, a sample is drawn, typically at 150 ml min^{-1}, from a connector at the patient's airway and carried via a narrow catheter to the analyser. A moisture trap is present as shown and the analyser has an exhaust port which allows the gas to be returned to the patient's breathing system, for example when a fully closed breathing system is in use. Alternatively, the exhaust gases may be channelled to the theatre scavenging system. In the side-

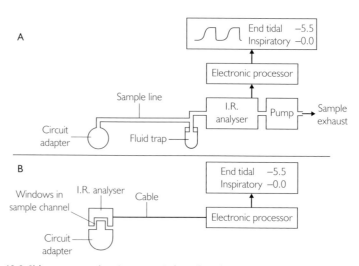

Figure 19.6 Side-stream and main-stream infrared analysers

stream system, the transit time for the sample to move along the catheter will delay the overall response time of the analyser, but if the correct tubing and flow is used, this time will be less than 1 s and no serious modification of the signal is incurred.

In the main-stream system, a special connector is needed in the breathing system and it incorporates a channel with sapphire windows. The analyser sits over this channel as shown and the infrared beam passes directly through the gases in the airway. In this way a sampling line is avoided and the transit time is nil. The connector is, however, bulkier than in the side-stream system.

Some instruments only provide an indication of the end-tidal carbon dioxide concentration, but most anaesthetists now prefer to have a full capnograph trace (Fig. 19.7). Apart from information from the shape of the trace, knowledge of its baseline can be valuable, as a rise of baseline could indicate a failure of some component such as a valve in the breathing system. A sudden change of the capnograph pattern to a straight line gives the anaesthetist prompt warning of failure of the ventilation or of the patient's circulation, for example due to an air embolus. A progressive rise of end-tidal carbon dioxide may indicate inadequate ventilation or the onset of malignant hyperpyrexia.

For accuracy a capnograph needs a rapid response time. This time has two components: the transit time and the rise time. The transit time is the time for the sample to be transferred to the analyser and, as indicated earlier, the transit time of the side-stream analyser is normally not important as the signal is only delayed and not seriously distorted. The rise time represents the time for the analyser to respond to the signal and is so called from a test procedure in which a step (i.e. sharp) change of sample concentration is arranged and the time measured for the indication on the analyser to change from 10% to 90% of the final value. The rise time will depend upon the size of the sample chamber and the gas flow. A short rise time of under 400 ms and good signal reproduction is obtained by use of a small analysing chamber, e.g. 1 ml, but it is important that the appropriate flow is used. Too low a flow will give an unacceptably long rise time. Too high a flow can also give incorrect results because it could cause a significant pressure drop across the sampling line and the output of the analyser depends on pressure.

In addition to its use for carbon dioxide measurement, the infrared analyser may also be used for nitrous oxide and other anaesthetics. A special application is its use for trace concentrations in the atmosphere. To achieve the additional sensitivity in this case, a long infrared beam is needed because there are then more infrared absorbing molecules lying in the beam. One way to lengthen the beam is to have a longer sample cell but this would necessitate a larger sample and a slow response time. In practice this problem is solved by the use of angled mirrors to fold the beam so it passes a number of times through the sample. Such folded beam instruments are still large and have a comparatively long response time but can detect gases in concentrations of a few parts per million. Consequently, they can measure trace anaesthetic concentrations in the atmosphere.

Figure 19.7 Recording of expired carbon dioxide tension

The carbon dioxide electrode and the infrared analyser are the principal techniques for analysing carbon dioxide, but gas chromatography and mass spectrometry (Chapter 20) may also be used.

In the colorimetric technique, the change of [H+] when a dye is exposed to carbon dioxide leads to a change of colour. This can be used to give warning of the expiry of soda lime used in closed circuits.

Gastric Mucosal pH

Failure of the liver or kidneys may take place when blood is diverted to organs such as the heart and brain as an early response to a threatened circulation. The diversion of blood through the process of splanchnic vasoconstriction results in hypoperfusion of the gut. It is thought that when blood flow falls below the minimum value that is necessary to meet metabolic demand, carbon dioxide accumulation and acidosis results and that this affects the mucosa. Bowel wall hypoperfusion may result in tissue injury, increased permeability, easier movement of bacteria and endotoxins, and a harmful inflammatory response. The adequacy of splanchnic oxygenation and blood flow may therefore relate to the prognosis of critically ill patients and may be assessed through the measurement of gastric mucosal pH (pHi).

Gastric pH is measured with a nasogastric tonometer. A gastric tonometer catheter is used, which is a nasogastric tube with an additional channel connected to a sealed balloon. The tube is impermeable to gas but the silicone balloon is permeable. The balloon lies within the stomach lumen and is inflated with several millilitres of saline or air. Over a period of time, the carbon dioxide pressure within the balloon equilibrates with that in the lumen of the stomach and, in turn, with the pressure in the gastric mucosal cells. If the arterial bicarbonate concentration is known, the carbon dioxide tension in the samples withdrawn from the balloon can be used to calculate the intracellular pH by means of the Henderson–Hasselbalch equation:

$$pH = pK + \log_{10} \frac{[HCO_3^-]}{[H_2CO_3]} = pK + \log_{10} \frac{[HCO_3^-]}{\alpha \, PaCO_2}$$

where pK is the negative logarithm to the base 10 of the equilibrium constant for the disassociation of carbonic acid and α is a proportionality constant relating the concentration of arterial carbonic acid to the arterial PCO_2. Values below 7.32 indicate intracellular acidosis, reflecting inadequate oxygen delivery.

In one form of automatic tonometer, a pump automatically transfers air to and from a tonometric balloon every 10 min. The sample is transferred to an analyser working on the infrared principle. The air is recycled to the catheter balloon to avoid carbon dioxide depletion in the catheter system, thereby decreasing subsequent equilibration times. This provides automated measurement of gastrointestinal carbon dioxide tension ($PgCO_2$).

If a double-lumen catheter is used, gas can be recirculated continuously, providing a measurement with a response time of about 5 min.

Further Techniques of Gas and Vapour Analysis

20

In addition to the usual methods of gas and vapour analysis considered in previous chapters, there are several other less commonly used techniques that may be employed.

Gas Chromatography

Chromatography literally means to write in colour. As shown on the left of Fig. 20.1, if a mixture of dyes is poured into a column packed with calcium carbonate, the pigments separate out as coloured bands at different levels and the components may eventually be collected from the outlet. Chromatography is now a general term for analytical procedures that separate a mixture into its components as the mixture passes through a column. The calcium carbonate in the example forms a stationary phase which retains the individual dyes for different periods, hence separating the mixture. The dye mixture passing through forms a mobile phase.

In a gas chromatograph there is also a stationary phase and a mobile phase, as shown on the right of Fig. 20.1. The stationary phase, with which the chromatographic column is packed, usually consists of a support material such as silica-alumina in the form of very small particles which is then coated with polyethylene glycol or silicone oil. Through the column containing this packing passes a flow of carrier gas, such as nitrogen, argon or helium, which forms the mobile phase. The gas mixture to be analysed is injected into the inlet of the column into the mobile phase and the components pass through the column at a speed which depends on their differential solubility between the two phases. The term gas–liquid chromatography (GLC) is sometimes used for this system. As solubility is temperature dependent, the column is maintained at a preset temperature in a thermostatically controlled oven (Fig. 20.2).

As shown in Fig. 20.2, the column is usually a long coiled glass tube containing the packing material. The added length of the column gives better separation of the components. A flow control provides a steady stream of carrier gas, in this case nitrogen, through the column and an injection port for the sample is provided at the column inlet.

Detector

At the outlet of the column, a detector is connected to a recorder to monitor the appearance of the sample components. A typical example is the flame ionization detector (Fig. 20.3).

In the flame ionization detector, hydrogen and air are added to the gas to produce a flame at the end of the column. The constituents of a flame are ionized particles. If a polarizing voltage is applied across the flame by two electrodes, a current is produced. The magnitude of this current depends on the particular

Figure 20.1 Principle of liquid chromatography (left) and gas chromatography (right)

Figure 20.2 Gas chromatograph

Figure 20.3 Flame ionization detector

Figure 20.4 (A) Thermal conductivity detector, (B) electron capture detector

charged particles in the flame. If a sample of organic vapour is present in the carrier gas, it is ionized in the flame and increases the current flow. The size of the current increase gives a measure of the amount of organic vapour present.

As shown in Fig. 20.3 the gas chromatograph recording appears in the form of a peak as each component of the sample passes out of the column.

There are two main alternatives to the flame ionization detector: the thermal conductivity detector (also called the katharometer), and the electron capture detector. The katharometer (Fig. 20.4A) measures changes in thermal conductivity of the gas by the change in the electrical resistance of a heated wire placed in the gas flow. It is more suitable than the flame ionization detector for the analysis of inorganic gases such as nitrous oxide or oxygen.

Halogenated compounds can be detected with greater sensitivity by an electron capture detector (Fig. 20.4B). In this detector, a polarizing voltage is applied across an ionization chamber in which electrons, released from a radioactive cathode, constitute a flow of current to the anode. Halogenated compounds from a sample capture these electrons and reduce the current flow.

None of these detectors allows the absolute identification of the unknown components of a sample, and it is necessary to have preliminary knowledge of the types of substances present and to apply this knowledge to the analysis of the recorder tracing.

Analysis of the Recorder Tracing

As different pure substances progress at characteristic rates through the separation column, the time between the injection of a sample and its appearance at the detector may be used to identify the component. This period is known as the retention time, and is 4 min in the example given in Fig. 20.3. In practice, a mixture of substances may be present in the sample and several peaks, each with its characteristic retention time, appear on the tracing (Fig. 20.5).

Provided that the nature of the sample components is known, calibration samples of known quantities of these can be injected, as shown in Fig. 20.5. These allow confirmation of the presence of the substances, and the comparison of the

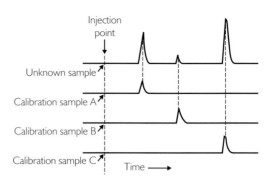

Figure 20.5 Comparison of the chromatograph peaks from a sample with those of calibration samples

peak heights (or, more accurately, peak areas) permits calculation of the quantity of each substance.

Introduction of a Sample into the Gas Chromatograph

The sample is usually injected as rapidly as possible from an appropriate gas-tight syringe through a rubber septum. If the port at which the injection is made is heated, then injected liquids are vaporized and the volatile components may be analysed. In this way, even blood samples can be analysed directly in a gas chromatograph. As an alternative to the use of a gas-tight syringe, gas samples may be introduced by a special gas-sampling valve.

Clinical Use

Gas chromatography is used for measuring volatile anaesthetic agents, both for anaesthetic concentrations and for trace levels in the theatre atmosphere. The gas chromatograph is also of use in the measurement of barbiturates, phenothiazines, benzodiazepines, steroids and catecholamines, special techniques being used to convert these into volatile compounds.

Gas chromatography has several advantages in that it allows the identification and measurement of very low concentrations of drugs, even in a mixture of compounds; the technique is versatile in that both liquids and gas samples can be analysed. However, its disadvantages are that continuous analysis is impossible and details of the sample constituents must be available.

The Mass Spectrometer

References are made in other chapters to the use of the mass spectrometer to measure water vapour, oxygen and carbon dioxide, but this instrument can also be used to separate and measure other gases. The sample is drawn through a tube into the sample chamber of a mass spectrometer by a pump. As illustrated in Fig. 20.6, a molecular leak permits a few molecules of the sample to diffuse into an ionization chamber where they are bombarded by a beam of electrons passing from the hot cathode to the anode. This beam of electrons is produced in the same way as in the oscilloscope. When the molecules of the gas are hit by the electrons, some of them become charged ions which are then accelerated out of the chamber in a narrow beam by means of the acceleration and focusing plates. The stream of ions

Figure 20.6 Principle of the mass spectrometer

then passes through a strong magnetic field. The charged ions are deflected in an arc by the magnetic field. The amount of deflection depends on their mass: the lighter ions are deflected most and the heaviest least. In Fig. 20.6 four different ion streams are shown, only one of which passes through a small slit to be picked up by a detector. The signal from the detector depends on the number of ions reaching it, and this signal can be amplified and displayed. By varying the voltage on the acceleration and focusing plates, the position and speed of the beam may be altered and streams of ions of different masses detected.

Another method (Fig. 20.7) of picking out specific streams of ions uses four electrically charged rods in place of the magnetic field. The potentials on the rods are varied so that the ions oscillate between them as they travel. It can be arranged so that only ions of a specific mass are able to travel the length of the rods without being removed from the stream. This system is known as a quadrupole mass spectrometer.

Although the mass spectrometer identifies compounds by their mass numbers, many molecules fragment during the ionization process. For example, the introduction of carbon dioxide into a mass spectrometer results in the detection of carbon dioxide, carbon monoxide and oxygen ions, having mass numbers of 44, 28 and 16, respectively.

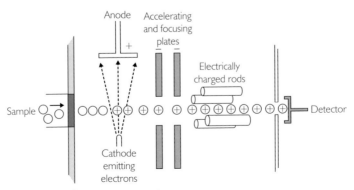

Figure 20.7 Quadrupole mass spectrometer

If a mass spectrometer is used to analyse a gas mixture, a large number of ions is produced and some of the ions have the same mass number. The concentration of a particular component of the gas mixture can be determined by choosing an ionized fragment of the compound of interest which has a different mass number from any of the other ions present. An example of this is the analysis of nitrous oxide in the presence of carbon dioxide, as both have the same mass number of 44. The nitrous oxide fragments on ionization, and the smaller nitric oxide fragment with a mass number of 30 can be identified and used to measure the concentration of nitrous oxide. A detailed knowledge of the cracking patterns, i.e. the ratios in which fragments are produced, can help in the identification of components in a gas mixture.

The mass spectrometer is a versatile instrument which may be used to measure many different gases and compounds. In anaesthesia, mass spectrometers with a rapid response time of less than 100 ms have been used for breath analysis of expired air. Because the mass spectrometer can identify compounds and analyse very small samples, it is also used in isotope studies and in conjunction with gas chromatography.

Other Techniques of Vapour Analysis

Although the gas chromatograph and mass spectrometer are highly versatile instruments, they are bulky and less convenient for use in areas outside the laboratory. Anaesthetists often use alternative techniques in such areas.

The solubility of anaesthetic agents in certain types of material is the principle used by one form of anaesthetic vapour analyser. When an electric potential is applied across a crystal of quartz it contracts slightly: this is known as the piezo-electric effect. The crystal can be made to oscillate at its resonant frequency by a suitable alternating potential, and the vapour analyser uses such a crystal to which a thin coating has been applied. Anaesthetic agents dissolve in the coating and alter the resonant frequency of the crystal. From Henry's law, the quantity of vapour which dissolves is proportional to the partial pressure of the vapour, so the change in resonant frequency of the crystal can be measured electronically and displayed as anaesthetic concentration. The analyser is not specific to individual anaesthetic agents, and responds to a limited extent to water vapour. Nevertheless, the analyser forms a useful instrument for measuring anaesthetic vapour concentration: for example, in the closed circuit.

Anaesthetic vapour concentration can also be measured by the infrared analyser described in Chapter 19 (Fig. 19.5) and by the refractometer. The refractometer is an appropriate instrument for analysis of individual samples and for checking the performance of vaporizers; its principle is described in Chapter 13.

Other techniques which have been used for gas analysis include the measurement of the velocity of ultrasound in a gas mixture and the application of Raman spectrometry.

Raman Effect

Electromagnetic radiation can interact with a molecule in several ways. The radiation may simply be scattered by the molecule, after which the energy of the scattered radiation is the same as the energy of the incident radiation but the radiation is travelling in a different direction. Alternatively, there may be a transfer of energy between the radiation and the molecule, which results in a change in the energy possessed by the molecule. The molecule may absorb the energy of the incident radiation completely (this is the process occurring when infrared light is used to measure carbon dioxide partial pressure, for example), or there may be a partial transfer of energy between the radiation and the molecule. This latter process is known as the Raman effect. In the Raman effect, the energy transfer affects the energy of vibration associated with bonds between atoms in the molecule, so absorption of radiation at a particular wavelength is associated with a specific type of bond between atoms in the molecule.

Since the energy of radiation is proportional to the frequency of the radiation, the transfer of energy between the radiation and the molecule results in a change in the wavelength of the radiation. Although the molecule can transfer energy to the radiation, the reverse process – the transfer of energy from the radiation to the molecule – is much more common, so the effect usually observed is a decrease in the wavelength of the radiation. The decrease in wavelength is a characteristic of an individual type of molecule, so the Raman effect can be used to measure the partial pressures of a range of gases of interest in anaesthesia.

The Raman effect is a comparatively weak effect, so an intense source of light, typically a laser, must be used to generate enough Raman radiation to achieve a measurable signal at a detector. The detector must not be in line with the incident radiation as it would be impossible to identify the low-intensity radiation resulting from the Raman effect in the presence of the incident radiation. The axis of the detector is therefore usually perpendicular to the axis of the source of radiation.

The working principles of one type of anaesthetic gas monitor that uses the Raman effect are shown in Fig. 20.8. A helium–neon laser is used as the source of radiation, a sample cell being included between two mirrors at either end of the light path from the laser. There is a set of eight detectors, only two of which are shown in the figure. Each detector comprises a filter that allows radiation of a specific wavelength only to pass and a photodetector that converts incident radiation to an electrical signal for subsequent measurement and processing. The filters are manufactured to pass Raman radiation characteristic of oxygen, nitrogen, carbon dioxide, nitrous oxide, the C–H bond and three volatile anaesthetic agents. The three volatile anaesthetic agents to be analysed are specified when the instrument is purchased and the appropriate filters are installed by the manufacturer. The sample is drawn into the chamber through a type of tubing that removes water vapour, so that a dry sample is analysed.

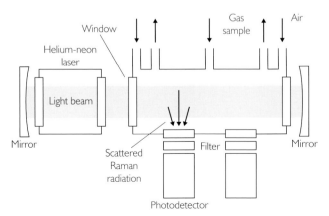

Figure 20.8 Gas analyser based on the Raman effect

The signal from the photodetector measuring the radiation arising from the C–H bond is used to measure the concentration of volatile anaesthetic agents, as, although this signal arises from several different agents, there is usually only one present at a time and the signal is stronger than the signal that can be obtained from other bonds within such molecules. The signals from the photodetectors that respond to the Raman radiation from the individual volatile agents are used to determine which agent is present. If more than one volatile agent is present in the sample chamber at the same time, the C–H bond detector is still used to measure the total Raman radiation arising from the volatile agents, but the relative concentrations of the agents are obtained from the detectors measuring the radiation from the individual agents. Because the signals from the individual agent detectors are weaker than the signal from the C–H bond detector, the result is less accurate than when one volatile agent is present.

The intensity of the radiation beam generated by the laser is capable of degrading volatile anaesthetic agents. To avoid any resulting compounds being deposited on the windows of the sample cell, thus reducing its measuring efficiency, air is pumped past the cell windows to shield them from contact with the sample and any degradation products.

Gas Supplies

21

The maintenance of medical gas supplies and the care of medical gas cylinders are usually under the supervision of a hospital's engineering and technical staff, but anaesthetists using gas supplies and cylinders should have some knowledge of the topic.

Gas Cylinders

Most large gas cylinders are stored in the upright position, but some smaller ones and Entonox cylinders are stored horizontally. Cylinders should be stored indoors, protected from the weather and should not be subjected to extremes of heat or cold; they should also be used in rotation with separate areas for full and empty cylinders. Cylinders containing medical gases should be stored separately from other types and separate areas should be allocated for flammable gases such as cyclopropane. To withstand high pressure, the cylinders are made of high carbon steel, manganese steel or aluminium alloy, although even these steels will not prevent the risk of an explosion if the cylinder is dropped on a hard concrete surface.

Cylinders are identified not only by clear written labels but also by colour coding. In the international standard of colours for medical gases (ISO/R32), oxygen cylinders are black with a white top, nitrous oxide blue, cyclopropane orange and carbon dioxide grey. The international system is adopted in the UK, but in the USA and some other countries different colour codes may still be seen.

Around the neck of a cylinder in the UK is a plastic disc, the colour and shape of which denotes the year when the cylinder was last examined (Fig. 21.1). The manufacturers regularly examine and test cylinders, including an internal examination with an endoscope, so that any faulty ones may be withdrawn from use. The interval between testing varies but is usually from 5 to 10 years, depending on the gas.

On the top of the cylinder is an identification label summarizing safety precautions. There are risks of explosion and fire if oil or other flammable liquids are allowed to come into contact with high-pressure oxygen, nitrous oxide or Entonox, since all these gases support combustion.

Heating cylinders is dangerous because it increases the pressure inside them. A moderate rise in temperature as occurs in summer, however, is not important, because the cylinders are made to withstand pressures well above their normal working range. The actual value of the pressure that the cylinder can withstand depends on its type and on the gas concerned, but it is usually 65–70% above the working pressure.

The cylinder valve should be opened momentarily before attaching the cylinder to the anaesthetic machine. This blows out any dust or other material which might be lodged in the outlet of the cylinder and which might otherwise enter the anaesthetic apparatus.

Figure 21.1 Gas cylinders – pin index system and test discs

After attaching the cylinder, it is recommended that the valve is opened slowly to avoid adiabatic heating (Chapter 4). It should be opened two full turns because valves that are only partially open may restrict the flow of gas when the cylinder pressure falls. Finally, only moderate force should be used when closing the valve as otherwise the valve seating can be damaged.

Figure 21.2 shows a detailed section of the valve seating. A spindle with a plastic facing is screwed up and down against the valve seating. This plastic facing may be damaged if the valve is closed too tightly. Around the spindle, below the nut at the top, is a compressible plastic washer known as a gland which prevents any leak while still allowing the spindle to turn.

On the face of the valve block are holes which correspond with pins on the yoke of the anaesthetic machine. This arrangement comprises the pin-index system, a device to prevent connection of the wrong cylinder to the yoke of the anaesthetic machine. There is a special pin-index configuration for each medical gas; Fig. 21.1 illustrates the configuration for oxygen, Entonox and nitrous oxide.

Instead of the pin-index system, there are two other systems used on the larger cylinders. A large bull-nose cylinder, typically used for oxygen, is shown on the left

Figure 21.2 Section through a cylinder valve

Figure 21.3 Thread patterns for larger cylinders

Right-hand screw for non-flammable gases but left-hand screw for hydrogen

of Fig. 21.3. It has a right-hand internal thread on the cylinder outlet identical to that used for the large air, helium and nitrogen cylinders. For hydrogen and other flammable gases, however, the cylinder outlet has a left-hand thread, giving some protection against wrong connection.

On the right of the diagram, the valve of a large nitrous oxide cylinder is shown. Notice that it has an external thread connection and may also have a hand-wheel. Similar handwheel cylinders may also be seen outside the UK, often containing other gases but with different patterns of thread. These systems, however, give only partial protection against incorrect connection.

Piped Oxygen Supplies

To avoid frequent changing of cylinders of gases in busy theatres and for reasons of economy, gases may be piped from a remote storage area. The most common piped supply is that of oxygen and the central source may be a cylinder manifold or a liquid oxygen tank. However, in either case the oxygen storage area should be outside or not in direct communication with the main hospital buildings, because there is an increased fire risk in all areas where oxygen is stored.

In many hospitals the oxygen supply is in the form of a cylinder manifold; Fig. 21.4 shows such a manifold with its cylinders attached. The six cylinders illustrated are divided into two banks of three and are so arranged that each bank contains the correct number of cylinders to last for a minimum of 2 days' normal use; hence, the size of the manifold varies according to the size of the hospital.

Figure 21.4 Oxygen manifold

In Figure 21.4, the three cylinders on the left are in use, the three on the right in reserve. Each cylinder is connected by a coiled tube to a pipeline which passes to a central control box. The high-pressure gauges on the left and right sides of the box indicate the contents of the cylinder banks, and below are high-pressure reducing valves which reduce the cylinder pressure of 137 bar to about 10 bar. The changeover valve, shown in the centre, has a pneumatic shuttle mechanism which is held at its extreme positions magnetically, but which switches automatically from the bank of cylinders in use to the bank in reserve when the pressure falls to a certain value. Electric warning devices are provided, and are activated by the changeover shuttle valve. These may switch on warning lights or audible alarms, both at the control box and at remote points, to indicate the need to change the empty bank of cylinders. A secondary fail-safe bypass system with additional cylinders may also be present to ensure a continued supply even in the event of a changeover failure.

At the outlet of the shuttle valve is a second-stage reducing valve to reduce the pressure from 10 bar to 4.1 bar, the normal pipeline pressure. A pressure gauge for monitoring purposes is present and there may also be an alarm that operates if excessively high or low pressure develops. Pressure relief valves are present to prevent high pressure developing in the pipeline.

The main source of piped oxygen in large hospitals is not from cylinders but from a liquid oxygen supply. The underlying principle of the liquid oxygen supply is discussed in Chapter 10. This supply usually has a capacity to last for at least 6 days but there is also a reserve manifold of cylinders. A control mechanism operates between the liquid oxygen supply and the bank of cylinders so that if the liquid supply fails for any reason, this mechanism automatically turns on the cylinder supply.

Entonox Supplies

Oxygen is not the only gas which may be piped to theatres and intensive care areas from a central source. Entonox, nitrous oxide and air may also be supplied from a manifold of cylinders.

Entonox is a mixture of 50% oxygen and 50% nitrous oxide, stored in gaseous form in cylinders at a pressure of 137 bar. If a full cylinder of Entonox is cooled, a liquid phase, containing about 20% oxygen and 80% nitrous oxide, may form below the gas (Fig. 21.5).

Figure 21.5 Effect of cooling below −5.5°C on an Entonox cylinder

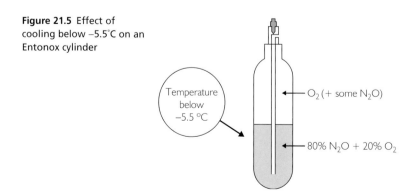

Temperature below −5.5 °C

O_2 (+ some N_2O)

80% N_2O + 20% O_2

Depending on the pressure in the cylinder, this may take place at a temperature as high as −5.5°C. If the gaseous phase is drawn from a cylinder in which this condensation has occurred, the gas initially contains a high percentage of oxygen. However, the oxygen concentration falls as the oxygen passes out of the liquid phase to replace that drawn from the gaseous phase. Eventually, both the liquid and gas phases contain very little oxygen. To prevent this occurring, large cylinders have a dip tube which draws off any liquid phase first. This prevents the delivered oxygen concentration falling below 20% at any time. Nevertheless, this is only a secondary safety provision and it is recommended that the temperature in the storage area for these cylinders is maintained above 10°C.

The nitrous oxide manifold is very similar to the oxygen manifold. In this case, the cylinders contain liquid nitrous oxide and so have a greater reserve of gas than the equivalent oxygen cylinders.

Compressed Air Supplies

Air is another supply often piped to theatres and, although it can also be provided from a manifold of cylinders, a central compressor plant is a more economical source for larger hospitals.

Figure 21.6 illustrates the main components of a central compressor plant. In practice, apart from the reservoir, the main units are duplicated so that any item can be serviced or repaired without interrupting the air supply. The air intake shown on the top left should normally be out-of-doors in such a position that it is not affected by rain, snow, dust or fumes. Air from the intake is drawn through a preliminary filter and a silencer into the compressor, which incorporates an after-cooler to cool the air once it has been compressed. The air then passes via a non-return valve into the large cylindrical receiver, which acts as a reservoir to maintain a constant air pressure.

After leaving the reservoir, the air is cleaned by means of separators and filters and then dried before it is piped to the theatres and wards. Most compressors are oil-lubricated; consequently, it is essential that oil mist is removed from the compressed air so that patients breathing it do not get oil pneumonitis. Coarser droplets of oil are baffled out in the separators; then finer particulate matter is

Figure 21.6 Compressed air supply and central vacuum supply systems

removed in the filters. The air too must be dried because its relative humidity will have increased on compression. Two driers are present in each unit and they contain a suitable desiccant material such as silica gel. They are fully automatic and change from the drier in use to the reserve should the air humidity rise. The humidity should be such that the dew point of the air supplied is less than −40°C.

A final filter follows the drier to ensure an air supply free of bacteria. The actual distribution pressure of the air is higher than for other piped gases; it is usually 6.9 bar because the piped air is commonly used to operate surgical tools. Alternatively, separate air supplies for surgical tools and for anaesthetic use may be provided.

Centralized Vacuum System

A centralized vacuum system is another supply often installed as part of a medical gas pipeline system and, as with the piped air supply, the vacuum system consists of a pump, a large receiver and a filter unit, as shown in Fig. 21.6. In the bottom right of the figure is the typical vacuum terminal unit through which the air from wards and theatres is first drawn into drainage traps and bacterial filters to dry and clean it. The air then passes into a cylindrical receiver which acts as a reservoir to maintain a constant suction; this also prevents the duty pump having to run continuously when the load is light. One pump is illustrated but there are normally two, each of which is capable of maintaining a vacuum of not less than 0.67 bar (500 mmHg) below the standard atmospheric pressure of 1.01 bar (760 mmHg). The exhaust gases from the pump pass through a silencer before being discharged out-of-doors, usually away from windows or other air intakes. In some hospitals an active scavenging system for anaesthetic gases may be used which works on the same principle as the vacuum supply but usually without a vacuum reservoir.

Suction Apparatus

Suction apparatus is connected to the vacuum pipeline; Fig. 21.7 illustrates a typical suction control. Application of a vacuum through the inlet evacuates the compartment below the diaphragm. The setting of the control knob at the top alters

Figure 21.7 Suction control system

the pressure of the spring on the diaphragm. This in turn varies the pressure at which the diaphragm control valve opens or closes the inlet, so adjusting the degree of vacuum. The vacuum is indicated by a gauge. Below the control valve is a compartment with a float control and a filter; a collection jar with its own float control lies between this compartment and the patient. The two float controls protect the suction control system and the pipeline by occluding the airflow if the compartments become full and the filter provides additional protection from particulate and nebulized matter.

Although general purpose suction units may provide an unrestricted flow greater than 25 litres min^{-1} and a vacuum greater than 0.67 bar (67 kPa), vacuums and flows as great as these are not suitable for all purposes and can be dangerous if used in an inappropriate application. Drainage of a closed cavity, for example, must be carried out with a low vacuum and a low flow.

The Oxygen Concentrator

The oxygen concentrator has some similarities to the central compressor plant used to provide compressed air, but in addition incorporates cylinders containing zeolite. This is a silicate compound which has ion-exchange properties and acts as a molecular sieve, separating the oxygen from nitrogen in the air. It is similar to materials used to pack some chromatographic columns.

Figure 21.8 illustrates the principle of its action. As in compressed air supplies, the air is filtered, then compressed and cooled before being dried by silica gel. However, in addition to the silica gel, the two cylinders shown also contain the zeolite, which absorbs nitrogen. Solenoid valves direct the flow of gas so that one cylinder absorbs nitrogen and water vapour while absorbed gas from the other is drawn off by the vacuum pump. The solenoid valve reverses every half minute to give a steady flow of oxygen-enriched air to the reservoir.

Small oxygen concentrators are available for use in the home for long-term domiciliary oxygen therapy. They can give oxygen concentrations of 90–95% and a flow of 4 litres min^{-1}, and are more convenient than oxygen cylinders. The running cost, which includes electricity and servicing, is much less than that of cylinder or liquid oxygen supplies. Although 2–5% argon is present in the oxygen mixture produced by concentrators it appears to have no toxic effect. The balance of the gas delivered is mainly unabsorbed nitrogen and carbon dioxide.

Figure 21.8 Oxygen concentrator; C is the cylinder containing zeolite and S is the solenoid valve

A disadvantage of these concentrators is that the oxygen concentration delivered can decrease with increasing flow: the flow is usually restricted to a maximum of about 4 litres min^{-1} and the maximum pressure available is often about 70 kPa. This pressure is much lower than the 410 kPa provided from cylinder reducing valves and by the piped gas supplies in hospitals, so if ventilators and equipment using venturis have been designed for hospital use, they may be unsuitable for use with the smaller oxygen concentrators. However, larger oxygen concentrators are made for small hospitals and clinics in remote areas lacking reliable oxygen supplies, and these provide the gas at a higher pressure and flow.

Piped Medical Gas Outlets

All the piped medical gas supplies to theatres and other areas finish in special terminal units with a non-interchangeable coupling; in the UK, this is a type of Schraeder valve and is illustrated in Fig. 21.9. The non-interchangeability is achieved by the use of various sizes of collar on the probe so that a given collar only fits the appropriate outlet; thus, the nitrous oxide collar has a larger diameter than the oxygen collar, as shown. Outlets are also labelled and colour coded and contain an internal valve which seals the gas supply until the probe is plugged in. On unplugging, the valve closes off the gas supply.

Leaks and Faulty Connections

A leak at any point in the gas supply system or at the anaesthetic machine is a matter for concern. If a leak occurs at the pin-index mounting point it could indicate a fault at the non-return valve, which is usually incorporated between the cylinder and the reducing valve. Alternatively, it could be due to damage to a Bodok seal, the compressible washer present at this point. Leaks at other points in the anaesthetic machine may result in the patient receiving less gas than intended and may also cause an increase in air pollution in the theatre.

Leaks can also occur if connections in the anaesthetic tubing systems are not secure; connections are available with a screw collar to provide a more secure lock, as shown in Fig. 21.10.

Great care is needed not only to avoid leaks but also to prevent any risk that anaesthetic system tubing or gas supply leads are connected incorrectly.

Suppose, for example, that unauthorized personnel have wrongly connected the nitrous oxide and oxygen tubings on the anaesthetic machine as shown in Fig. 21.11. The anaesthetist may not notice this immediately if using mixtures of oxy-

Figure 21.9 Piped medical gas terminal units

Figure 21.10 Screw collar system for use with anaesthetic tubings

Screw collar

Figure 21.11 Risk of reversal of oxygen and nitrous oxide supply leads

→To patient

O_2 N_2O

O_2

N_2O

gen and nitrous oxide, but it may result in the patient being awake during anaesthesia and in an emergency the patient may receive 100% nitrous oxide instead of 100% oxygen with fatal consequences.

Figure 21.12 illustrates the rapidity with which the alveolar oxygen tension falls if a pure anoxic gas such as nitrous oxide is administered to the patient. In 5–10 s a dangerously low alveolar oxygen tension (PAO_2) is achieved, followed almost immediately by a drop in the arterial oxygen tension (PaO_2). This fall is much more rapid than in the case of respiratory obstruction because when breathing is obstructed there is a reserve of oxygen in the lungs, whereas in the case shown in Fig. 21.12 the oxygen is being actively washed out of the patient's lungs and blood.

This problem may also occur if the oxygen supply fails or is allowed to run out while the nitrous oxide supply continues; modern anaesthetic machines now incorporate safety warning devices and a nitrous oxide supply cut-out to protect the patient in the event of oxygen supply failure (Chapter 1).

Repairs to Piped Gas Supply Systems

In addition to accidents caused by errors with the gas supply at the anaesthetic machine, problems have arisen when repairs have been made to the piped gas supplies.

A repair to an existing pipeline which involves depressurizing and altering the pipeline is classed as a major hazard repair. If maintenance or repairs are carried

Figure 21.12 Fall of alveolar oxygen tension during ventilation with an anoxic gas

out on a piped medical gas system, it is important that the terminal units affected are not in use at the time and that certain tests are carried out at every outlet before the system is put back into service.

Medical air is used to carry out a leak test in which the whole system is pressurized and sealed. Over a period of 24 hours there must be no unacceptable drop in pressure. An anticonfusion test is performed by connecting medical air to one pipeline system at a time and ensuring that the test air is delivered from every terminal unit bearing the name of the gas pipeline system being tested but is not delivered from any other terminal unit.

Repairs to pipelines can cause particulate contamination in pipes so purging at each affected gas outlet is required to remove loose particles in the pipeline and to ensure that the pipeline contains only gas from the supply. Purging involves opening the valve at each outlet fully for a period of about 4 min. This test may cause a rapid reduction in the gas pressure in the pipeline system and may activate the associated alarms. For this reason all theatre and other relevant staff should be informed when gas testing is to be carried out.

Particle testing involves passing the gas from selected outlets through a filter at a rate not less than 150 litres min^{-1} for 30 s and then checking the filter for particles.

After the pipeline systems have been connected to their appropriate gas sources, tests must be carried out to check the identity and purity of the gases delivered at the terminal units. An oxygen analyser is used to check the identity, giving readings of 0% for nitrous oxide, 21% for air, 50% for Entonox and 100% for oxygen. A chemical gas detection tube may be used to test the purity of the gas delivered and to detect any impurities which may have been introduced into the system by pipe jointing procedures. One pipe jointing procedure involves filling the pipe for a few feet either side of the join with carbon dioxide to reduce oxidation while the pipe is heated. The carbon dioxide is removed by purging, but each affected outlet must be tested for carbon dioxide afterwards and must not deliver more than 300 ppm.

Air from a compressed air supply should be tested further to ensure that it is free from impurities such as water, oil, carbon monoxide and carbon dioxide.

These procedures are primarily the responsibility of the hospital authorities but anaesthetists should have a general knowledge of them so that appropriate precautions are observed.

Breathing and Scavenging Systems

22

This chapter deals first with the systems by which gases or anaesthetic vapours may be delivered to the patient's airway.

The Open System

This is the simplest system and is illustrated in Fig. 22.1. In this system, the patient's airway remains open to room air and no tubing, valves or reservoir bag are used. In the first example, A, the anaesthetist is inducing anaesthesia in a child by allowing the anaesthetic gases to fall over the child's face from a cupped hand containing the end of the gas delivery tube. In earlier forms of anaesthesia, a Schimmelbusch mask was used, held over the patient's face in a similar manner. In example B, oxygen is delivered to an Edinburgh mask which has a wide opening to room air and produces a negligible increase in the respiratory dead space. In example C, oxygen is delivered by cannulae to the patient's nostrils. A similar technique has also been used during anaesthesia, a constant flow of anaesthetic gases being delivered by the side tube of a special gag into the mouth of the patient.

Open systems have the advantage of presenting no added resistance to the patient's breathing, but the disadvantage of giving little control over the concentration of oxygen and other gases received by the patient, because air dilution is inevitable. During peak inspiration, a large inspiratory flow of up to 50 litres min^{-1} may occur, so dilution with air is high during this part of the respiratory cycle.

Known concentrations of gases can only be administered if the flow of gas to the patient exceeds the peak inspiratory flow. Some oxygen therapy Venturi masks achieve this by the use of an injector technique (Chapter 2).

To administer more accurately controlled concentrations of gases, a tightly fitting face mask or intubation is used. The main breathing systems may be categorized as non-rebreathing valve, T-piece, Magill and closed systems. All the systems have a reservoir in the form of tubing or a bag to allow adequate gas supply to the patient during peak inspiratory flow.

Non-Rebreathing Valve Systems

A typical non-rebreathing valve is the 'Ambu E' valve, illustrated in Fig. 22.2A. It contains moulded rubber one-way inspiratory and expiratory valves positioned to allow the patient to draw in gas through one connection and expire through the other. In the example shown, a reservoir bag is present in the system and the gas supply to this must equal the tidal ventilation.

The Ambu E valve can also be used for controlled ventilation, as shown in Fig. 22.2B. Squeezing the reservoir bag applies positive pressure to the inspiratory port, moving the valve flap to occlude the outlet as shown. Thus, the Ambu E valve can act both as an inflating valve and as a non-rebreathing valve. In a variety

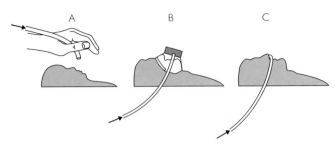

Figure 22.1 Open breathing systems

of the valve, the Ambu E2, used only in resuscitation apparatus, the expiratory flap valve is omitted and the non-rebreathing function is then no longer present. It is important that these two types of valve are not confused, particularly when they are reassembled after cleaning. Valves should be closely supervised in use lest an excessive flow of fresh gas maintains the valve in the inflation position (Fig. 22.2B), resulting in a dangerous increase in airway pressure.

Because the pressures needed to overcome the inspiratory and expiratory valve resistances can be 100–200 Pa (1–2 cmH$_2$O) during peak flow, many non-rebreathing valves are uncomfortable for long-term use in conscious individuals. In breathing apparatus used for airmen, firemen and divers, non-rebreathing systems have special low-resistance flap valves and the Entonox apparatus used for analgesia has a similar low-resistance expiratory valve. In place of the inspiratory valve a special demand valve is used for Entonox, as described in Chapter 1, and similar demand valves are used to deliver air or gaseous mixtures in breathing apparatus.

A non-rebreathing valve system is useful for emergencies outside hospital, as it allows anaesthesia to be administered even when cylinder gas supplies are not available. Figure 22.3A illustrates one such system, the Triservice apparatus. Inspiratory and expiratory valves are incorporated in the Laerdal valve and, as in the Ambu E, the inspiratory valve can also function as an inflating valve (Fig. 22.3B). Thus, the silicone rubber flaps of the valve occlude the expiratory ports when the self-inflating bag is compressed. Air is drawn through a Triservice vaporizer, which is a modified OMV (Oxford Miniature Vaporizer, Chapter 11), and the T-junction shown allows oxygen supplementation should supplies be available.

Figure 22.2 Non-rebreathing system with Ambu E valve: (A) during expiration, (B) during positive inspiration

Figure 22.3 Triservice apparatus: (A) during expiration and (B) during positive pressure inspiration

The advantages of this system are its extreme lightness and portability. Similar systems are also possible with other draw-over vaporizers.

T-piece Systems

The T-piece system is sometimes known as Ayre's T-piece, after Dr Philip Ayre, who first used it in infants in 1937. There are no valves in the simplest form of this system. Fresh gas is supplied to a T-piece at the patient, who breathes through an open limb of the T-system, as shown in Fig. 22.4. This limb must be of suitable diameter to avoid excessive resistance to the flow of gas: e.g. 22-mm internal diameter for an adult patient.

In a typical system, a fresh gas flow of 2–2.5 times the tidal ventilation (e.g. 14 litres min^{-1}) is supplied to the T-piece and the capacity of the open limb could be the same as the patient's tidal volume. The figure illustrates the content of the open limb at the end of expiration, when it contains a mixture of expired and fresh gas. The gases from the patient's anatomical dead space are expired first, so these are shown released from the open end of the tube at A. During mid-expiration, the majority of the alveolar gases are expired at near-peak expiratory flow, so they are only slightly diluted by the fresh gas flow, as shown in the centre of the tube at B. At the finish of expiration, the expiratory flow falls, so the end of the tube nearest

Figure 22.4 T-piece system; gas distribution towards the end of inspiration (see text)

Fresh gas 14 l min^{-1}

the patient, C, contains more fresh gas. If there is an end-expiratory pause, a further volume of undiluted fresh gas is finally present, as at D in the figure.

Consider now what happens during inspiration. Initially, fresh gas only is inspired until inspiratory flow becomes greater than the flow of fresh gas to the T-piece. At peak inspiration, the patient may in addition draw upon the gas at D in the open tube. Provided there is an end-expiratory pause, this is fresh gas, so no rebreathing of alveolar air occurs.

If the fresh gas flow is too low, e.g. below twice the tidal ventilation, the patient will draw upon the gases at B and C in the open limb during peak inspiration and rebreathe alveolar gases.

Figure 22.5 illustrates the effect of the end-expiratory pause upon the fresh gas flow required to prevent any rebreathing of alveolar gas. The graph shows the gas volume inspired from the open limb of a T-piece by an anaesthetized patient with a tidal volume of 0.4 litre, breathing at a rate of 12 breaths per minute. The respiratory cycle therefore lasts 5 seconds.

The difference in the vertical height between the inspired gas volume and the fresh gas volume supplied is the volume of fresh gas in the open limb. If at any time the volume of inspired gas exceeds that of fresh gas supplied and stored in the open limb, rebreathing will occur. It can be seen from the graph that a flow of 14 litres min^{-1} (2.9 times the given tidal ventilation) is necessary if there is no end-expiratory pause. Provided that an end-expiratory pause of 1 s is present, then a flow of fresh gas of 8.5 litres min^{-1} (just under twice the tidal ventilation of 4.8 litres min^{-1}) ensures that the volume of fresh gas supplied always exceeds the volume of inspired gas from the open limb.

At the T-piece, the patient inspires from the fresh gases as well as from the open limb, so this limb need not be as large as the full tidal volume. Nevertheless, if the open limb is omitted, this leads to inspiration of air unless the fresh gas flow is equal to the patient's peak inspiratory flow.

It is possible to add an open-ended reservoir bag (Fig. 22.6A), or a bag with a valve to the open end of the T-piece (Fig. 22.6B). Movements of the bag indicate respiration and the bag can be used to control ventilation. When the T-piece is used with controlled ventilation, it is possible to use lower fresh gas flows because tidal ventilation can be increased to compensate for the rebreathing of alveolar gas

Figure 22.5 T-piece system; effect of an end-expiratory pause on the fresh gas flow required to prevent rebreathing of expired alveolar air (see text)

Figure 22.6 T-piece system: (A) with bag and (B) with bag and valve

from the open limb. In this case too, the pattern of ventilation can be adjusted to give an adequate end-expiratory pause to render the system more effective.

The T-piece system is particularly suited to use in paediatric anaesthesia because the T-piece connection can be close to the patient's airway with negligible apparatus dead space at this point. In addition, in its simplest form, it avoids the problems associated with an expiratory valve, such as increased resistance to flow and possible malfunction due to sticking. In adults, a disadvantage of the system is the high fresh gas flow which is required during spontaneous breathing. Apart from the cost, the added flow increases expiratory resistance and may increase the risk of pollution from spilt gas.

Coaxial T-piece System

A coaxial T-piece system is a more compact form in which the gas delivery tube of the T is inside the limb of the T (Fig. 22.7). Typical examples are the Bain (USA) or Penlon coaxial (UK) systems. As in other T-piece techniques, gas flows during spontaneous breathing should be about 2.5 times the patient's tidal ventilation. Special care is needed in these systems to ensure that the central tube carrying fresh gas is correctly attached, otherwise the fresh gases may not be delivered to the patient end of the tube.

Figure 22.7 Coaxial T-piece system

Magill System

The Magill system (Fig. 22.8) was introduced by Sir Ivan Magill in 1920. It comprises a reservoir bag, delivery tube and expiratory valve and remains a popular system for administration of anaesthesia in a spontaneously breathing patient. The figure illustrates the contents of the tube at the end of expiration. Gases from the anatomical dead space travel along the tube at A, while fresh gas inflates the reservoir bag, distending it until the pressure from the bag is sufficient to open the expiratory valve: this could be at 50 Pa or 0.5 cmH$_2$O pressure. Gases from the patient's alveoli are then expired through the expiratory valve into an expired gas scavenging system, or released into the atmosphere. Because the Magill system can conserve the dead space gas, it can be used at fresh gas flows of 70% of the patient's tidal ventilation in a spontaneously breathing patient.

The Magill system can also be used to ventilate the patient, the expiratory valve being tightened to a suitable extent and the reservoir bag squeezed to give intermittent positive pressure to the limits set by the valve. Excess gas spills from the valve at the end of inspiration. Because the gas spilt in this case is mainly fresh, the system is inefficient during controlled ventilation, but may be convenient for short-term use while an alternative, e.g. a ventilator, is arranged.

Modern expiratory valves are larger than the former 'Heidbrink' type expiratory valves, as they incorporate a connection for a scavenging tube. However, if the bulk of the valve is inconvenient, it can be positioned remote from the patient, as shown in Fig. 22.9A. A Magill system with remote valve can be convenient if it is decided to use disposable tubing to achieve better sterility, as the valve need not then be changed with each fresh tubing.

Coaxial Magill System

The coaxial Magill system also uses a remote expiratory valve, as illustrated in Fig. 22.9B. In the system shown, known as the Lack system, the fresh gas flows from the reservoir bag through the wide tube which contains a narrower tube leading to the expiratory valve. Unlike the coaxial T-piece, the patient breathes through both tubes in the coaxial Magill system. Hence, wider coaxial tubes are required to prevent increased resistance to breathing. The same precautions must be taken as in other coaxial systems to ensure that the internal tube is correctly fitted and positioned. As in the case of the standard Magill system, the coaxial Magill is less suitable for prolonged controlled ventilation.

Figure 22.8 Magill system: gas distribution towards the end of expiration

Figure 22.9 (A) Magill system with remote expiratory valve, (B) coaxial Magill system

Closed Systems

In the fully closed system, also known as the closed circuit or circle system, the patient's gases recirculate through soda lime, which absorbs carbon dioxide, while oxygen is added to replace the patient's metabolic uptake. A typical arrangement is illustrated in Fig. 22.10, but the positions of the components may vary.

The soda lime used must have granules of a critical size, large enough to avoid excess resistance to breathing and small enough to absorb carbon dioxide efficiently; a typical size is '4–8 mesh', indicating that the granules will pass through

Figure 22.10 Circle system; when fully closed, the fresh gas flow is oxygen at a rate equivalent to the patient uptake, with additional anaesthetic vapour as required; the reservoir bag illustrated can be replaced by a calibrated spirometer to indicate volume changes

a sieve having four strands per inch, but not through one with eight strands per inch.

When the system is used for anaesthesia, anaesthetic vapour is added in the concentration needed to meet clinical requirements and the uptake by the patient. The anaesthetic may be supplied from a draw-over vaporizer in the circle (VIC), or by an out-of-circle vaporizer (VOC). The latter needs to be a special type which retains its accuracy at low flows. Because of the variability of the patient's uptake of oxygen and anaesthetic agents, gas analysers are recommended when the closed system is used. This is to ensure that the concentrations of oxygen, carbon dioxide and anaesthetic vapours are satisfactory.

Other problems include the difficulty of sterilization because of the size and complexity of the closed system compared with the simpler versions, and the need for a special form of ventilator. The closed system has the advantage that it allows the oxygen uptake at the patient to be monitored, and the uptake of volatile anaesthetic agents to be demonstrated. Furthermore, the heat loss from the patient is slightly reduced because the inspired gas is fully humidified at near ambient temperature (Chapter 10). The economy in the amount of volatile anaesthetic used must be balanced against the added cost of the soda lime required. Another advantage, the reduction of pollution, is less relevant now that scavenging systems are recommended.

If a fresh gas flow of, for example, 2 litres min^{-1}, is supplied to the closed system and excess gas spilt from the expiratory valve, the concentrations of gases in the system approximate to those in the fresh gas supply. This system, sometimes described as a closed system with leak, gives better control of the concentrations but lacks some of the advantages claimed for the fully closed system.

If nitrous oxide were to be used with a fully closed system, the presence of nitrogen in the system would prevent the build-up of an adequate concentration of nitrous oxide. The use of a closed system with leak, at least for the initial period of use, allows the nitrogen to be replaced by nitrous oxide.

Alternative Classification of Systems

Unfortunately, there is no international standard for the classification of breathing systems. Even the word 'system' is not universal as some use the word 'circuit' instead. Nevertheless, the term 'system' is preferred in the classification given here, as only in the closed system does the breathed gas complete a circuit.

In the UK, systems such as the Magill, which are neither closed nor open, are often referred to as 'semi-closed'; however, in the USA, the term 'semi-open' is used instead, the term 'semi-closed' being used for the closed system with leak. In view of this confusion, the terms semi-open and semi-closed are best avoided.

Following an analysis of the performance of some breathing systems by Mapleson, the letters used by him to identify systems are as follows:

- T-piece system (unmodified)   E
- T-piece system with open-ended bag F
- T-piece system with bag and valve   D
- Magill system   A

The systems B and C in this classification are now seldom used and are not described in this chapter. The open, non-rebreathing valve and closed systems are not included in this categorization.

Resistance of Breathing Systems

The open system gives no added resistance to breathing, but in other systems, resistance occurs in the tubing and valves used.

If the tubing diameter is large enough to allow laminar flow, the additional pressure needed to overcome the resistance during inspiration and expiration is very small. As explained in Chapter 2, the critical flow for a smooth tube of 22 mm internal diameter carrying a mixture of nitrous oxide and oxygen could be about 22 litres min^{-1}. Anaesthetic systems use corrugated tubing and peak flows may exceed 22 litres min^{-1}, so both laminar and turbulent flow usually occur during the breathing cycle. Nevertheless, the extra pressure the patient must generate to drive the gases through the tubing is small – perhaps about 25 Pa (0.25 cmH$_2$O) during peak flow.

In patients having respiratory investigations involving the breathing of air or oxygen mixtures, even this small pressure may be undesirable, so tubing of a larger diameter, e.g. 30 mm, is used. Because laminar flow resistance is inversely proportional to the fourth power of the radius, the increase of diameter from 22 mm to 30 mm gives a 3.5 times reduction in resistance to laminar flow. In addition, the increased diameter reduces the risk of turbulent air flow which would give a sharp increase in resistance.

In simple T-piece systems without any expiratory valve or reservoir bag, the resistance is that of the limb of the T through which the patient breathes. In practice, the pressure required to be generated by the patient to overcome this resistance is greater during expiration than during inspiration. This arises because expiratory flow is increased by the fresh gas flow, whereas inspiratory flow in the limb is reduced by the fresh gas flow. The higher the fresh gas flow, the greater will be the back pressure during expiration. This factor applies generally in most breathing systems.

The valves are an important source of resistance in other breathing systems. A typical valve may have an opening pressure of 50 Pa (Chapter 1). However, during peak flows of about 30 litres min^{-1}, the turbulence in the valve results in higher pressures of 100–500 Pa (1–5 cmH$_2$O), depending upon the valve concerned.

The reservoir bag used in a system can also affect the pressures which develop during spontaneous breathing.

Work Used in Breathing Systems

The additional work required in breathing systems can be indicated by the area of a pressure–volume loop (Chapter 8). Figure 22.11 illustrates the type of loop for various systems. The pressure at the patient connector is plotted against the volume change for a tidal volume of 0.4 litre.

As explained above, the main source of resistance is in the valves of a system. Therefore, the simple T-piece system gives very little added work, as shown by the small area of the loop in Fig. 22.11A. In the case of the non-rebreathing valve or circle system (Fig. 22.11B), or the Magill system (Fig. 22.11C), the mean pressure swing could be 200 Pa (2 cmH$_2$O) for the volume change of 0.4 litre. The area of the loop and the work done during one cycle of ventilation would then be as follows:

$$\text{Additional work done} = 200 \text{ Pa} \times 0.4 \times 10^{-3} \text{ m}^3$$

$$= 0.08 \text{ J}$$

$$= 80 \text{ mJ}$$

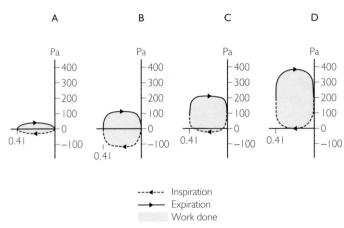

Figure 22.11 Work in breathing systems; graphs of the pressure change at the patient's airway for a tidal volume of 0.4 litre (spontaneous ventilation); (A) simple T-piece system, (B) non-rebreathing valve or circle system, (C) Magill system and (D) T-piece with reservoir bag and valve

The total mechanical work for a normal inspiration could be 300 mJ, so a typical breathing system could give a 27% increase in the work of breathing. Such increases of work are uncomfortable for conscious individuals but, as already explained, special valves with lower resistances are then used.

In the anaesthetic non-rebreathing valve system, the resistances of the inspiratory and expiratory valves are comparable, so the pressure–volume loop illustrated (Fig. 22.11B) shows that the inspiratory and expiratory work are similar, as indicated by the equal areas above and below the zero pressure axis. A circle system would give a similar result.

In the Magill system, there is no inspiratory valve and the assistance to inspiration from the slightly distended reservoir bag and from the fresh gas flow overcomes the small flow resistance of the 22-mm diameter tube. Consequently, all the work required from the patient to overcome the system resistance occurs during expiration, and it is seen (Fig. 22.11C) that the pressure–volume loop is almost entirely above the zero pressure axis. The coaxial Magill system performs similarly, but the expiratory resistance in this case is that of the valve with its central 12.5-mm diameter supply tube.

The T-piece system with a bag and valve could give a similar tracing if gas flow were comparable, but a high fresh gas flow of 2–2.5 times tidal ventilation is recommended. In consequence, the mean expiratory flow through the valve and tubing is increased, and much higher pressures are generated in expiration, as shown in Fig. 22.11D. The high gas flow maintains a positive pressure during part of an inspiration, assisting this phase of the cycle, so the patient uses less energy during inspiration. A similar tracing could be obtained with the coaxial T-system.

In anaesthesia in a spontaneously breathing patient, if the increase in the work of breathing required with a system is excessive, it may augment the depression of ventilation which occurs. The added expiratory resistance gives a slight rise in intrathoracic pressure and so could reduce venous return and cardiac output.

Because a face mask rarely gives a completely airtight fit, a system which raises the mean inspiratory pressure inside the mask has the advantage that air dilution of the anaesthetic gases during inspiration is reduced. During expiration, on the other hand, the leakage of the gases round the mask increases if the mask pressure is raised, and so air pollution is increased.

Safety of Breathing Systems

The components of breathing systems must be correctly assembled and there should be no risk of the connections falling apart accidentally. Couplings with screw collars are available and these should prevent unintentional disconnections (Chapter 21). However, the final connection at the patient is normally a simple cone fitting to allow rapid change of this coupling as needed. Plastic connections may distort during autoclaving and even metal ones can be damaged by misuse, so regular inspection is recommended with replacement as necessary. The security of push fit connections depends on an adequate area of contact between the tapers of the two connectors, so couplings which do not fit properly should not be used. A taper gauge can be used to test the dimensions of connectors against the appropriate standard.

Breathing tubes should not be too narrow and sharp angles at connections should be avoided as they not only increase the incidence of turbulent flow but also the resistance to breathing (Chapter 2).

Grossly excessive pressures can arise if the expiratory valve sticks or if it is omitted from the breathing system. Alternatively, excess pressure can build up if the scavenging tubing is obstructed. In such cases, the pressure builds up to the limit governed by the reservoir bag, if one is present. This pressure depends on the tension T in the wall of the bag and on the radius R according to Laplace's law:

$$P = \frac{2T}{R}$$

When the bag is distended, the tension in its wall due to its elasticity is proportional to the circumference of the bag, and this in turn is directly proportional to the radius. Hence, the bag gives a pressure that is nearly constant, even though it becomes grossly distended.

This pressure is usually about 4 kPa (40 cmH$_2$O) and this gives some short-term protection to the patient while the anaesthetist identifies and removes the obstruction in the system.

Some disposable reservoir bags lack elasticity and give no such protection, so pressures in the system then rise to much higher values. If the system lacks a reservoir bag entirely, then the pressure may rise to the limit set by the safety valve on the anaesthetic machine. Typically, this could be 35 kPa. Such a valve protects only the mechanical components of the machine and gives no protection to the patient.

In connecting any breathing system, the T-connection, or in the standard form of Magill system the expiratory valve, must be positioned close to the patient's airway so there is no excess anatomical dead space. An example of an accidental increase of dead space arises if the central tube of a coaxial system becomes detached. The entire coaxial tube may then be added to the dead space and the patient may suffer hypoxia and hypercapnia in consequence.

Ventilators

A full description of ventilators is beyond the scope of this book. However, as an example, Fig. 22.12 shows in simplified form the principle of a ventilator of the Manley Pulmovent type.

Figure 22.12 Simplified diagram to illustrate the principle of a ventilator of the Manley Pulmovent type; the ventilator is shown at the start of inspiration with both control ports of the cycling valve open

A fresh gas flow of, for example, 7 litres min^{-1} inflates a reservoir bellows. The gas in the bellows is at a pressure of about 10–12 kPa due to the force exerted on the bellows by springs. When the bellows are inflated to the preset volume, the cycling mechanism opens a valve to allow the bellows to inflate the patient's lungs. The full pressure of 10 kPa is not however applied, as a flow control valve restricts the flow as shown and a safety valve at the patient's side of the cycling valve limits pressure to a maximum of 7 kPa. The cycling valve also controls the expiratory valve, so this valve is closed during inspiration and open during expiration. During expiration, the airway is open to the atmosphere through the expired gas port while the reservoir bellows re-inflates.

It is convenient to classify ventilators as 'constant-pressure generators', in which the gas is supplied at a constant pressure during inspiration, and 'constant-flow generators', in which gas is supplied at constant flow. However, the Manley ventilator exemplifies a general problem in this classification in that, although a near-constant pressure is generated, it is applied via a flow control, so that neither pressure nor flow is constant at the patient's airway.

The cycling valve is tripped through levers by the tidal volume in the bellows, a control allowing the volume to be adjusted to meet requirements, so it might be regarded as a 'volume cycled' ventilator. However, clear-cut classification of the cycling of ventilators is also fraught with difficulty, as the volume delivered from the bellows is supplemented by the fresh gas flow in this case. The total minute volume is the fresh gas flow delivered from the anaesthetic machine, which is 7 litres min^{-1} in the example; so, if the tidal volume is 0.5 litre, the ventilation rate is 14. Thus, the ventilator is sometimes referred to as a minute volume divider.

Figure 22.12 also shows the two controls needed to convert the ventilator to a system for manual control or spontaneous breathing. One control bypasses the reservoir bellows and cycling valve so the fresh gases are delivered directly to the patient, while the other control bypasses the expiratory control valve, replacing it with a reservoir bag and expiratory valve. The breathing system is thus converted to a T-piece system. Some forms of Manley Pulmovent ventilator also incorporate an extra bellows to give a facility for negative pressure during expiration.

To reduce the possibility that a disconnection of the breathing system, a failure of the gas supply or the development of excessive pressure in the breathing system will pass unnoticed, it is advisable to use a ventilator alarm which monitors the pressure in the breathing system and gives a warning if this pressure either exceeds or fails to reach preset limits. A ventilator alarm usually has two adjustable pressure sensors. One sensor is set to the maximum pressure desired in the breathing system and operates an over-pressure alarm immediately this pressure is exceeded. The other sensor is set at a suitable pressure below the peak inspiratory pressure and operates a cycling alarm if the interval between occurrences of the set pressure exceeds about 15 s. This alarm may therefore detect disconnection of the breathing system or failure of the gas supply through decreased end-expiratory pressure.

Scavenging

An increased incidence of spontaneous abortion has been reported in female staff employed in operating theatres and early reports suggested that this might be due to exposure to trace quantities of anaesthetic agents in room air. Despite the fact that subsequent studies have not substantiated this suggestion, it is still reasonable to reduce the level of pollution by scavenging the expired anaesthetic gas.

Systems can be classified as active, in which an external source of power such as a pump draws away the scavenged gas, or passive, in which gases are driven to the exterior of the building by the pressure generated by the patient during expiration.

Like breathing systems, the simplest technique for active scavenging is an open technique, sometimes referred to in Scandinavia as 'local scavenging'. Other techniques of anaesthetic gas scavenging are more complex and British Standards are specified according to the system used for the transfer, receiving and disposal of the gases.

Open Scavenging Technique

In this technique, the point at which suction is applied to the waste gases is open to the atmosphere without any intervening reservoir bag or valves. The technique is generally less effective than the other systems. Techniques have been tried in which a funnel is positioned near the expiratory valve and mask (Fig. 22.13A) to aspirate spilt anaesthetic agents, e.g. in anaesthesia for dental extractions in which an airtight mask fit is difficult to achieve. Alternatively, the funnel can be inverted in the form of a dish and used to collect gases released from the end of a T-piece breathing system. In a patient in the recovery area or after Entonox analgesia, the gases released from the airway may be scavenged by a funnel positioned close to the mouth (Fig. 22.13B). Like the open breathing systems, the open scavenging systems lack control. A high scavenging flow is needed and the funnel must be very close to the point of release of the gases to be effective.

Component Systems of Standard Techniques

Figure 22.14 illustrates the component systems in the standard anaesthetic gas scavenging technique. The term 'transfer system' is used for the wide-bore 30-mm

Figure 22.13 Open scavenging systems; scavenging flow is indicated at S

Figure 22.14 Component systems of the anaesthetic gas scavenging technique

diameter tubing with its 30-mm male and female conical connectors which transfers the gases collected from the exhaust port of the anaesthetic breathing system or ventilator to the 'receiving system'. Typically, this latter system is an open-ended cylinder. Finally, the 'disposal system' exhausts the gases to the exterior of the building.

Receiving System

A typical receiving system incorporates an open-ended reservoir, as illustrated in Fig. 22.15A. The technique could use a simple T-piece as shown in Fig. 22.15B, but the reservoir, usually a cylinder, improves efficiency. It may incorporate channelling and the open end of the reservoir or 'air break' is an important safety feature. It is essential that the system is designed to prevent any risk of obstruction at this air break, otherwise excess negative or positive pressure could be applied to the patient's airway. The system is designed so the scavenging flow, typically 80 litres min^{-1}, removes all expired gas. A flow control and flow indicator are included.

In other receiving systems still in use, a reservoir bag and safety valves are used (Fig. 22.16): the valves prevent any risk of excess positive or negative pressure. The diagram also illustrates a simple disposal system.

Figure 22.15 Anaesthetic gas receiving system

Figure 22.16 Scavenging system with bag and valves; the system becomes a passive one if it is used without the injector illustrated

Disposal System

To dispose of the scavenged gases, some hospitals have used the same system as the centralized vacuum system described in Chapter 21, but an independent system is now recommended. This may incorporate a fan instead of a pump to remove the scavenged gases. Although a fan will generate less vacuum, this is not necessarily safer, as even a low vacuum will give obstruction and risks of pulmonary oedema if it is applied via the breathing system directly to the patient's lungs. The British Standard specifies stringent testing procedures to ensure that there is no risk of excess positive or negative pressure, even when faults occur in the scavenging system. Full details of the procedures are beyond the scope of this book but, as an example, they include a specification that the pressure at the exhaust port must not exceed 50 Pa (0.5 cmH$_2$O) when tested with a flow of 30 litres min^{-1} into the system. In addition to direct effects on the patient, pressure changes from faults in the scavenging system have also been found to give problems due to their effect on the functioning of the expiratory valve or the ventilator.

For individual use in areas where there is only a single anaesthetic machine, a single pump or even an injector powered by compressed air has been used. Oxygen, too, has been used to drive such a system but gives an increased fire risk and such systems may not meet current standards.

Passive Scavenging System

In the passive system, a wide-bore tube conducts the expired gases outside the building. This technique can give problems, as excessive positive or subatmospheric pressures may be caused by wind movements at the outlet. Furthermore, if the outlet is above roof level, as recommended to prevent re-entry of the scavenged gases to the building, then the weight of denser anaesthetic vapour such as nitrous oxide gives a back pressure in the patient's breathing system.

The collection system with bag and valves shown in Fig. 22.15 has been used without the injector as a basis for a passive scavenging system. To avoid the pressure problems due to air movement at the outlet of the passive system, the expired gases can be conducted to the exit grille used for the theatre ventilation. For this disposal system to work effectively, it is essential that the theatre ventilation exit flow is suitable, as flows in the ventilation ducts may vary and reverse flow is not unknown. The use of an exit grille is also inappropriate in theatres in which the ventilation recirculates the air.

Theatre Ventilation

Regardless of the scavenging system used, some spillage of anaesthetic vapours is inevitable: e.g. at the end of anaesthesia, at induction or when using a face mask. Efficient theatre ventilation – e.g. 15 air changes per hour – is therefore recommended in areas where volatile anaesthetics are used.

Fires and Explosions

23

General Principles

In a fire or explosion, a combustible agent or fuel combines with oxygen or another oxidizing agent to give reaction products and the release of energy (Fig. 23.1). Before the reaction can start, a small amount of energy known as the activation energy must be supplied. The energy produced in the reaction appears as heat energy, which increases the temperature of the mixture. Once the temperature exceeds a certain level, the reaction becomes self-sustaining, as the energy produced is then sufficient to supply the activation energy to propagate the reaction.

Figure 23.2 shows the reaction for cyclopropane. The activation energy could be provided by a small spark. Two molecules of cyclopropane combine with nine molecules of oxygen to give six molecules each of carbon dioxide and water, and energy is released. If the initial mixture contains two volumes of cyclopropane to nine volumes of oxygen, i.e. an 18% concentration of cyclopropane, all the cyclopropane and oxygen are used up and transformed into the product molecules, carbon dioxide and water. This concentration is known as the stoichiometric concentration:

The stoichiometric concentration of any combustible vapour and oxidizing agent is the concentration at which all the combustible vapour and oxidizing agent are completely used up.

The most violent reactions take place in stoichiometric mixtures. If the proportions differ from this mixture, the reaction is less violent and when one component is greatly in excess of the other, the mixture cannot be ignited at all. The limits outside which the mixture will not burn are known as the flammability limits.

Illustrated in Fig. 23.3 are the flammability limits for cyclopropane in oxygen and in air. The lower and upper limits in oxygen are 2.5 and 63%, respectively, and within these is the narrower range within which explosions may occur. The usual anaesthetic concentrations for cyclopropane are within these limits and therefore carry risks of explosion. As the speed at which the reaction spreads through a mixture depends on the proportions of fuel and oxygen present, a fire rather than an explosion is likely to occur at proportions nearer the flammability limits, as illustrated on the left of Fig. 23.4.

In such a reaction, the pressure is close to atmospheric (1 bar) and the temperature is several hundred degrees Celsius. For proportions near the stoichiometric mixture in oxygen, on the other hand, the reaction may spread faster than the speed of sound and when this occurs an explosion rather than a fire takes place. When a mixture explodes, the reaction can spread at eight times the speed of sound and generate pressures as great as 25 bar and temperatures as high as 3000°C. The violence of the reaction may be moderated by the presence of other molecules in a mixture.

Figure 23.1 Principle of combustion

Figure 23.2 Combustion of cyclopropane

Figure 23.3 Flammability limits of cyclopropane in oxygen and in air

Figure 23.4 Comparison of conditions in a fire and in an explosion

As shown in Fig. 23.3, the flammability limits of cyclopropane in air differ from those in oxygen. In normal anaesthetic practice cyclopropane burns but does not explode in air; the range of flammability is reduced and the stoichiometric concentration is altered to around 4%. The inert nitrogen molecules not only absorb some of the energy produced but also do not take part in the reaction. Hence, the reaction is much less violent.

Figure 23.5 shows the reaction in the stoichiometric mixture in air. The ratio of cyclopropane to oxygen is the same in this case, but there are four nitrogen molecules present for every oxygen molecule, so the mixture contains two volumes of cyclopropane and 45 volumes of air to give a stoichiometric concentration of around 4%.

Nitrous oxide is also an oxidizing agent. Nitrous oxide rapidly breaks down in the presence of the heat of a fire or explosion to release oxygen, giving a 33% oxygen mixture and releasing further energy:

$$2N_2O \rightarrow 2N_2 + O_2 + energy$$

An explosion can be more violent when nitrous oxide is present than with oxygen alone because, when a fuel burns in nitrous oxide, more heat is produced than when the fuel burns in oxygen.

Other Flammable Agents

Ether behaves in a similar fashion to cyclopropane, as illustrated in Fig. 23.6. At the top of the diagram are the lower and upper flammability limits of ether in oxygen – 2 and 82%, respectively – and the stoichiometric concentration in oxygen

Figure 23.5 Reaction in a stoichiometric mixture of cyclopropane and air

Figure 23.6 Flammability limits of ether in oxygen and in air (about 14%) at which there is a risk of explosion. Below are the flammability limits of ether in air. Like cyclopropane, ether does not explode in air but burns within the concentrations shown.

The concentrations of ether in oxygen used in anaesthesia are within the limits for an explosion risk and within the flammability limits for ether in air. A special risk may arise if liquid ether is spilt and produces a high concentration of ether vapour near the floor. The concentration of ether may approach the upper limit of flammability in air and if the ether were ignited, it could burn with what are known as 'cool flames'. These are invisible and, as the name implies, are at a much lower temperature than normal flames. When ether burns, carbon dioxide and water are usually formed, but in cool flames, the oxidation is only partial and the final products include acetic acid and acetaldehyde. The danger of cool flames is that they can transmit the risk of ignition to the anaesthetic breathing system.

Some anaesthetic agents normally considered nonflammable will burn if mixed in the correct proportions with oxygen or nitrous oxide, and if a sufficiently high temperature occurs to ignite the mixture. Thus, the lower limits of flammability for halothane and trichloroethylene are higher than those likely to be used in normal anaesthetic practice. Also, any sparks present are unlikely to be of sufficient energy to start the mixture burning.

Many anaesthetists now use only nonflammable anaesthetics, but this should not give rise to complacency because many other flammable agents may still be brought into the theatre area. Perhaps the commonest is ethyl alcohol or surgical spirit. A saturated vapour of alcohol in air at normal room temperature gives a 6% mixture.

As shown in Fig. 23.7, a 6% mixture is near the stoichiometric concentration in air and carries a high risk of burning; the risk is increased further if oxygen or nitrous oxide is present. Accidents have also occurred when liquid spirit on the patient's skin has ignited. The pale blue flames may not be readily visible and severe burns may occur before the accident is noticed. Fires have also occurred with alcohol when it has been used in nebulized form to sterilize ventilators.

In addition to alcohol, there are flammable substances that are not anaesthetic agents but may give rise to fire or explosion risks. Thus, methane and hydrogen may be present in the patient's gut and may be ignited by electrosurgery when the gut is opened. Ethyl chloride may be used as a local anaesthetic spray and ether may be used to degrease the patient's skin. In addition to these flammable agents, many other combustible materials such as paper, plastic drapes and dressings are found in theatre.

Pure oxygen under pressure results in exceptionally high fire and explosion risks. Hence, oil and grease must be avoided in any part of the compressed oxy-

Figure 23.7 Flammability limits of ethyl alcohol in air

gen supplies, and special precautions are necessary in the areas of oxygen mani-folds or liquid oxygen supplies.

Activation Energy and Ignition Temperature

In a mixture of a combustible agent and oxygen, the molecules are normally kept apart by repulsive forces. For the mixture to burn, the molecules must be brought close enough to react together (Fig. 23.8). One obvious way of doing this is to increase the speed with which the molecules collide; this may be accomplished by increasing the temperature of the mixture locally, either by a spark or some other source of heat. The temperature must be raised to a sufficient degree over a suffi-ciently large volume and the energy required to bring this about is the activation energy.

The temperature to which a mixture must be raised for combustion to start is known as the ignition temperature, which varies with the constituents of the potentially explosive mixture and the proportions of the components. At the stoi-chiometric concentration of many explosive mixtures, the ignition temperature is about 400°C, but mixtures of ether and oxygen can ignite at a temperature as low as 150°C. This could occur if the mixture were brought into contact with a hot surface. Electrosurgical equipment is also an obvious source of heat, and lasers (Chapter 24) too can ignite flammable materials.

Sparks may also provide the activation energy to initiate explosions. They are highly efficient in doing this, as, in contrast to a hot wire or naked flame, a spark concentrates the energy into a very small volume. Sparks with an energy as little as 1 microjoule (1 μJ) can activate an ether–oxygen explosion when these gases are present in stoichiometric concentrations: one microjoule is a tiny amount of energy, being the amount needed to raise the temperature of 1 millilitre of water one-fifth of one-millionth of a degree Celsius.

Spark energy depends on the voltage of the source. A standard laryngoscope has a low-voltage battery and no explosions have been reported when intubating

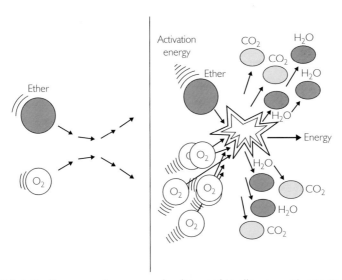

Figure 23.8 Activation energy increases molecular speed to allow a reaction to occur

patients using laryngoscopes in the presence of ether. In contrast, electrosurgical equipment uses high voltages. Even stray electrosurgery currents may cause sparks in the region of the patient's airway and anaesthetic connections and, consequently, flammable agents must never be used in the presence of electrosurgery. In X-ray departments, flammable agents are usually avoided because the possibility of sparks occurring in the X-ray apparatus cannot be eliminated. In this case full antistatic precautions, including an antistatic floor (see below), are not enforced because the cost is not justified.

Static Electricity

Static electricity is the other important source of electric sparks. To prevent the build-up of static electricity, the floors of operating theatres are electrically conductive to allow static charges to drain away. Too low a resistance is undesirable as it could increase electrocution risks, whereas too high a resistance would allow electrostatic charges to build up. To allow charges to be conducted to the floor, all apparatus and tables have conducting wheels or supports and staff wear antistatic rubber-soled shoes or clogs of the appropriate standard. Antistatic rubber contains carbon to make it electrically conductive and is also used for anaesthetic tubing. Materials with appropriate antistatic properties are also recommended for clothing and drapes: e.g. cotton is preferable to plastic. Endotracheal tubes, however, are not made of antistatic materials but are rendered conductive by the high humidity of the gases passing through them.

Equipment for Use with Flammable Mixtures

Equipment may act as a source of ignition for a flammable mixture if electric sparks are produced during its operation, if it produces static electricity or if parts of it reach high temperatures; nevertheless, equipment can be designed to avoid the ignition of flammable mixtures.

Flammable mixtures can be divided into two types: mixtures which contain oxygen or nitrous oxide as the oxidizing agent and mixtures which contain air as the oxidizing agent. Since the former need less activation energy for combustion to begin than the latter, it is possible to define two different zones of risk: a zone in which nitrous oxide or oxygen predominates as the oxidizing agent and a zone in which air predominates as the oxidizing agent.

A flammable anaesthetic mixture is normally contained within the breathing system and the patient's airways, and within anaesthetic apparatus and equipment attached to it, but may pass into the room air either as a discharge of expired gas or from a leak. In an unrestricted space it may spread up to 5 cm from the discharge or leak before becoming sufficiently diluted for air to predominate as the oxidizing agent. After the mixture has been diluted with air, it may remain flammable up to 25 cm from the leak or discharge. These two zones are shown in Fig. 23.9.

Flammable mixtures in which air is the oxidizing agent may also be formed near spirit-based preparations. The zones in which mixtures remain flammable can be modified or extended considerably if the source is extended, for example by the use of a spirit-based preparation applied over a large area, or if the space into which the flammable mixture disperses is confined, for example by drapes.

Equipment intended to be used in either of the two zones of risk must be designed and constructed according to principles that avoid sources of ignition.

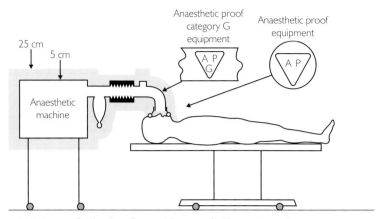

Figure 23.9 Zones of risk when flammable anaesthetic agents are in use

Two categories of equipment have been defined for use in the two different zones of risk:

- *Category APG equipment* is designed and constructed in such a way as to avoid the ignition of a flammable anaesthetic mixture with oxygen or nitrous oxide and is marked with the letters APG on a green band.
- *Category AP equipment* is designed and constructed in such a way as to avoid the ignition of a flammable anaesthetic mixture with air and is marked with the letters AP on a green circle. This equipment must not be used in a zone which contains a flammable anaesthetic mixture with oxygen or nitrous oxide.

Equipment which does not belong to either of these two categories may be marked as equipment not suitable for use in the presence of a flammable anaesthetic mixture with air, or with oxygen or nitrous oxide. However, if it is not indicated that equipment is category AP or category APG, it should be assumed in the absence of other information to be not suitable for use in the presence of flammable gas mixtures.

Isotopes and Radiation

24

Atomic Structure and Isotopes

An atom consists of a central nucleus containing protons that are positively charged and neutrons with no charge, and this nucleus is surrounded by orbiting electrons which have a negative charge. The type of atom, i.e. element, is determined by the number of protons (the atomic number); for example, hydrogen has 1 proton, carbon 6 and uranium 92. The neutrons contribute to the stability of the nucleus and, for a particular element with a given number of protons, different forms with different numbers of neutrons may exist. These different forms of the same element are called isotopes. An isotope of an element can be described by the total number of neutrons and protons which the nucleus contains, i.e. the mass number. Examples of isotopes include hydrogen-1, hydrogen-2 (deuterium) and hydrogen-3 (tritium); carbon-12 and carbon-14; and uranium-235 and uranium-238. Many isotopes of elements occur naturally, but others may be produced artificially in a nuclear reactor.

Isotopes are often described by a special method and the three isotopes of hydrogen – ^1_1H, ^2_1H and ^3_1H – are used here as an example: the superscript is the mass number and the subscript is the atomic number. The three isotopes of hydrogen are shown in Fig. 24.1.

The isotopes hydrogen-1 and deuterium are stable, but in the third, tritium, the nucleus is unstable and will not hold together indefinitely. Such an isotope is called a radioisotope, and is radioactive. The unstable nucleus of a radioisotope, also known as a radionuclide, eventually changes into another element in one of several ways. In the case of tritium, one of the neutrons in the nucleus changes into a proton and an electron; this electron is ejected from the nucleus (Fig. 24.2). The nucleus then contains two protons and one neutron, and the atom of tritium has changed into an atom of the stable element helium-3.

Modes of Decay

The process of one element changing into another is known as radioactive decay and may occur in one of the following ways:

- An electron, known as a beta (β) particle, may be emitted (as in the example above). Although an electron is negatively charged, a positively charged beta particle known as a positron may be emitted by some nuclei.
- The nucleus may capture one of the electrons surrounding it.
- An alpha (α) particle may be emitted. An alpha particle is a combination of two protons and two neutrons (i.e. a helium-4 nucleus).
- The nucleus may undergo spontaneous fission, i.e. splitting into several fragments.

Figure 24.1 Isotopes of hydrogen

These four options are not mutually exclusive and several types of decay may occur alternatively or in sequence.

After a nucleus has decayed by one of these processes, it is usual for the nucleus of the new element formed to emit one or more gamma (γ) rays. A gamma ray is not a particle but an electromagnetic wave (Chapter 13). However, because it has a high frequency and short wavelength, it behaves in many respects like a particle.

If there is a delay between the decay of the nucleus and the emission of the associated gamma rays, the nucleus is said to be in a metastable state until the gamma rays have been emitted. The metastable state has its own rate of decay or half-life (Chapter 5) and the metastable isotope is identified by an 'm' after the mass number, e.g. technetium-99 m.

The SI unit of radioactivity is the becquerel.

The Becquerel (Bq) A given quantity of radioactive substance has an activity of 1 becquerel if one disintegration of a nucleus takes place on average every second.

Formerly, radioactivity was defined in terms of the curie (Ci), where a curie is the quantity of any radioactive substance undergoing 3.7×10^{10} disintegrations per second.

Duration of Radioactivity, the Half-life

Radioactive decay is a random process, but the rate of decay at any moment will depend on the amount of radioactive isotope present; consequently, the process is exponential (Chapter 5). The rate of decay is measured by the half-life, i.e. the time required for half the radioactive atoms present to disintegrate. As an example, chromium-51 used in red cell volume measurement (Chapter 3) has a half-life of 27.8 days. Thus, if there are initially 10^{12} atoms of chromium-51 in a sample of a chromium compound, there will be 5×10^{11} remaining after 27.8 days. After a further 27.8 days there will be 2.5×10^{11} atoms of the isotope remaining, and so on.

Figure 24.2 Radioactive decay of tritium; the tritium nucleus decays to a helium-3 nucleus and a beta particle

Characteristics of Emitted Particles and Radiation

The alpha and beta particles and the gamma rays emitted by a radioactive isotope have a particular energy which is characteristic of the radioisotope concerned. The energy of electromagnetic waves is proportional to their frequency, and gamma rays and X-rays are also usually referred to in terms of their energy rather than their frequency. If the radioactive substance is within the body of the patient, all or part of this energy may be absorbed by the tissues. All the energy of alpha and beta particles is absorbed by the surrounding tissues, causing damage, but in the case of gamma rays, a proportion of the radiation escapes from the body and may be measured by a suitable detector. On the other hand, if a radioactive isotope emitting gamma radiation is outside the body, the gamma rays will penetrate the skin and be absorbed there and in the deeper tissues. A radioisotope can be sealed in a suitable container so that gamma rays only are emitted and any associated alpha and beta particles are absorbed in the container walls. Such sealed sources are used in the treatment of disease.

Alpha and beta particles and gamma radiation all cause damage to or death of cells. Actively dividing cells, such as tumour cells, are particularly vulnerable.

Detection of Radiation

Radiation may be detected using a scintillation counter, which is shown in Fig. 24.3. Gamma rays are absorbed in the sodium iodide crystal and their energy is converted into a flash of light. The intensity of the light is converted into an electrical pulse and amplified greatly by the photomultiplier tube.

The radioactivity in fluid samples containing isotopes which emit only beta radiation may be measured by mixing the sample with a liquid scintillator, which is a compound that will emit a flash of light when a molecule is struck by a beta particle. The flashes of light may then be detected and counted.

Therapeutic Uses of Radioisotopes (Radionuclides)

In the treatment of tumours, the radiation may be given by means of an external or internal source. At one time, cobalt-60, which has a half-life of 5.3 years, was used as an external source, but gamma rays are now generated externally by means of a linear accelerator. In some cases, an internal source of radiation is placed in the patient. Thus, a sealed yttrium-90 implant is used in the treatment of pituitary tumours which have caused acromegaly, and a sealed caesium-137

Figure 24.3 Scintillation counter

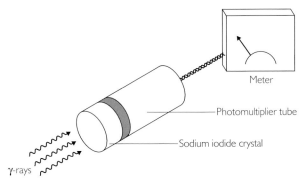

Meter

Photomultiplier tube

Sodium iodide crystal

γ-rays

capsule is implanted in the uterus in the treatment of some uterine tumours. Caesium-137 is also sometimes used with an 'after loading' technique. In this, cannulae are first placed in a tumour (e.g. of breast) and, once in position, caesium-137 needles are inserted down the cannulae to provide a high localized dose of radiation.

In addition to the therapeutic use of isotopes in the treatment of neoplasms, they are sometimes used to treat other conditions. Examples are the use of oral iodine-131 in the treatment of thyrotoxicosis or intravenous phosphorus-32 for polycythaemia rubra vera.

Diagnostic Uses of Radioisotopes (Radionuclides)

Diagnostic techniques using radioactivity may be divided into two groups: imaging and nonimaging.

Imaging Techniques

Imaging techniques use the gamma rays emitted from an isotope and an image of the distribution of a radioactive compound within the body can be obtained by using a gamma camera. The gamma camera is similar to the scintillation counter; the gamma rays interact with a large crystal of sodium iodide, causing the emission of flashes of light that can be detected electronically. From the positions of these flashes in the crystal, a picture of the isotope distribution in an organ may be built up.

Technetium-99m is the radioactive isotope commonly used in imaging techniques because it has the advantage of being easily attached to various chemical compounds which can be injected into the patient. It also has a short half-life of 6 hours, thus reducing the radiation dose to the patient, and it produces gamma rays of an energy suitable for forming a good image. Thus, technetium-99m labelled pertechnetate may be used for blood flow imaging and tetrofosmin for assessment of cardiac function, while labelled macroaggregated human serum albumin may be used in a lung scan to assess pulmonary circulation. Pertechnetate is also used for thyroid scans and exametazime for brain imaging. Other technetium labelled compounds are used for liver, bone and renal investigations.

An alternative form of lung scan uses either of the radioactive gases xenon-133 or krypton-81m. If a small quantity of one of these gases is inhaled, an image of its distribution allows the assessment of regional ventilation.

A different type of imaging technique has been used in experimental animals to investigate the uptake of anaesthetic agents. The anaesthetic agent is labelled with a radioisotope such as carbon-14 and after an animal has inspired the anaesthetic agent, it is sacrificed and sectioned. The sections are placed in contact with photographic film and, after development, the film is found to be darkened in areas due to exposure to the radiation from the carbon-14. An estimate of the relative uptake by various organs can then be made from the relative exposure produced on the photograph.

Nonimaging techniques

Nonimaging techniques using radioactivity include the use of chromium-51 labelled red cells or albumin for the measurement of red cell volume or plasma volume, respectively. A small known quantity of radioactive red cells or albumin is injected and, after a suitable interval, the dilution of the radioactive tracer in the patient's blood can be measured and from it the red cell or plasma volume can be calculated (Chapter 3).

The blood flow into or out of an organ can be measured if a radioisotope is used as an indicator. Suppose an organ contains a given quantity of a radioisotope at a particular time. The rate at which the radioactivity decreases in the organ depends on the blood flow and the volume perfused by this flow. The situation is analogous to the washing out of muddy bath water considered in Chapter 5, and a plot of radioactivity against time is a washout curve, from which the time constant and thus the blood flow may be determined.

Fibrinogen labelled with radioactive iodine-125 may be used to detect deep venous thrombosis. The labelled fibrinogen is injected intravenously into the circulation. Should a clot begin to form, fibrinogen is locally concentrated within the clot. A proportion of this fibrinogen is the radioactive fibrinogen, which may be detected by means of the gamma rays it emits. A portable scintillation counter moved along the deep veins in the legs will show a locally high reading above a blood clot. In this test, it is necessary to block the uptake of radioactive iodine by the thyroid by giving the patient a large dose of potassium iodide beforehand.

Stable Isotopes

As stable isotopes are not radioactive, they are difficult to isolate or detect and have few special uses in medicine. They can be identified by the mass spectrometer described in Chapter 20.

X-Rays

X-rays, like gamma rays, are electromagnetic radiation but are produced in a different way (Fig. 24.4). They are produced when a beam of electrons is accelerated from a cathode to strike an anode, usually of tungsten. A divergent beam of X-rays is produced, and a lead shield with a window in it is used to restrict the size of the beam. X-rays are used for imaging purposes and in the treatment of disease.

Radiation Safety

As alpha and beta particles, gamma radiation and X-rays may all cause tissue damage and chromosomal changes, it is important that exposure to them is kept

Figure 24.4 Production of x-rays

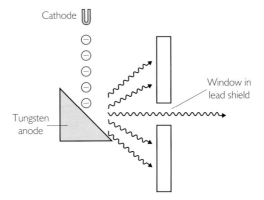

Cathode

Tungsten anode

Window in lead shield

to a minimum. An individual may be exposed to radiation from two sources: radioactive elements within the body and radioactive elements and other sources of radiation outside the body.

The ingestion of radioactive materials may be avoided by safe handling procedures designed to ensure that such materials are not allowed to contaminate surfaces where they are being used. Typical precautions would include the wearing of gloves by people handling the materials, and arrangements to contain spillage of radioactive liquids.

Exposure to external radiation may be reduced by enclosing radioactive sources in containers made of material that absorbs radiation. Alpha particles travel only a few centimetres in air before their energy is expended and therefore the principal problem is one of containment to ensure that no alpha-emitting material is inadvertently inhaled or ingested. Beta particles can travel a few metres in air before they are absorbed; hence, shielding a source with radiation-absorbing material is necessary. Because beta particles produce X-rays if decelerated rapidly, it is best to provide shielding with a material of comparatively low density, such as Perspex, to avoid unnecessary conversion of the beta-particle energy into X-rays. Gamma rays can travel large distances and shielding gamma-ray sources is best achieved with dense materials such as lead. A thickness of 7-cm lead will absorb at least 90% of gamma rays of the type emitted by radioisotopes. Lead also absorbs X-rays, so it is incorporated into aprons worn by staff exposed to radiation. Local shielding may also be used to protect parts of patients outside the main X-ray beam when radiographs are being taken.

As actively dividing cells are particularly affected by radiation, the fetus is at special risk even before the mother may realize that she is pregnant. It is thus recommended that, except in emergency, women of reproductive capacity should be X-rayed only in the first 10 days of their menstrual cycle, i.e. before ovulation has occurred (the 10-day rule).

Apart from the effects of absorption, the intensity of any radiation is inversely proportional to the square of the distance from the source. Hence, the dose of radiation received may be reduced greatly by moving away from the source.

Regular checks for contamination of surfaces where radioisotopes are used should be carried out; a scintillation counter may be used. Where it is not easy to predict what an individual's exposure to radiation will be or in circumstances where it is desired to check on the effectiveness of working practices, an individual may wear a photographic film badge to monitor the total radiation dose received. The film badge contains a small piece of photographic film behind several different filters and permits estimation of the energy and dose of radiation received.

Hospitals have available to them the services of a radiation protection adviser, who should be consulted before radioactive compounds are used; in the UK a doctor requires a certificate of authorization before being permitted to administer a radioactive compound to patients. The symbol shown in Fig. 24.5A is displayed when there is a risk of exposure to ionizing radiation.

Nonionizing Radiation

X-rays and gamma rays are known as ionizing radiations because their energy is dissipated in tissues initially through the process of the removal of electrons from atoms. The resulting ions are very reactive chemically, so that ionizing radiation is particularly hazardous. Radiation from other parts of the electromagnetic

Figure 24.5 Warning symbols for ionizing radiation (A) and lasers (B); the symbols are black on a yellow background

A   B

spectrum dissipates its energy in tissues in other ways, and is therefore known as nonionizing radiation.

Nonionizing radiation comprises radio waves, microwaves, infrared radiation, visible light and ultraviolet radiation. There are also hazards associated with the use of nonionizing radiation, so that protection measures must be considered for all types.

A special risk of burns from infrared or visible light radiation arises during the use of lasers. Lasers allow a beam of radiation to be focused onto a very small area, typically a spot of 0.1–2 mm diameter, depending upon the requirements. Lasers are used in ophthalmology, to treat retinal detachment or vascular diseases of the retina; in dermatology, to treat port wine stains; and in gynaecology, to treat neoplasms, e.g. of the cervix. In otolaryngology, lasers may be used to treat lesions in the mouth or of the larynx; they have also been used to remove tumours obstructing the trachea or bronchus.

In view of the safety hazards they present, the principle of the laser is considered in more detail.

Principle of the Laser

A laser produces an intense parallel beam of light or other electromagnetic radiation. An argon gas laser is shown in Fig. 24.6 and it can be seen that in some respects it is similar to a fluorescent light tube. In this laser, a high voltage is applied between two electrodes at the ends of a long narrow tube containing the gas. The current flow through the tube places the atoms of gas into a state in which they possess more energy than normal; this is known as an excited state. Excited states have a certain fixed energy difference from the normal or ground state. Consequently, when an atom returns from an excited state to the ground state, the energy is often dissipated as light or radiation of a specific wavelength characteristic of the atom.

The tube has windows at each end which are inclined to the path of the radiation at an angle known as the Brewster angle, the angle at which no internal reflection at the surface of the windows takes place; this ensures that 100% of the light is transmitted through the windows. The radiation is reflected back and forth along the length of the tube by mirrors at each end. The intense radiation inside

Figure 24.6 Principle of a gas laser

the tube causes the atoms to return to the ground state and emit radiation faster than would otherwise be the case. The radiation they emit is exactly in phase with the radiation already passing up and down the tube. The result is the conversion of the electrical energy into an intense, narrow, parallel beam of radiation which escapes from the tube through one of the mirrors which is partially silvered. It is this process which gives the laser its name, laser being an acronym for light amplification by stimulated emission of radiation.

There are numerous different types of laser and not all of them use gas. The lasing medium in the neodymium-YAG (yttrium aluminium garnet) laser, for example, is a solid rod in which the atoms are excited by a discharge lamp beside the rod.

The radiation from a laser has a specific wavelength; the argon laser, for example, produces visible light and is used in ophthalmology, whereas the carbon dioxide laser emits infrared radiation and is more powerful, being suited to surgical use when excision of tissue is needed. In some lasers, radiation is conducted along optical fibres to the point where treatment is needed. However, these fibres are opaque to the infrared radiation from the carbon dioxide laser, so its beam must be guided by a system of mirrors.

Optical Fibres

As mentioned above, optical fibres can be used with lasers to direct the beam, but they are also used in the design of endoscopes to permit a physician to see round corners. The principle of their action is as follows. The direction in which light travels is bent (refracted) as it passes from one substance to another with different optical properties (Fig. 24.7, top left). If the angle between the direction in which the light is travelling and the boundary between the two media is sufficiently acute, the light may be totally reflected (Fig. 24.7, top right).

An optical fibre is constructed from a core of glass or other transparent material, surrounded by a cladding layer. Reflection occurs at the boundary between the core and the cladding layer. Light passing into one end of an optical fibre can pass along the fibre by being continually reflected from the boundary between the core and the cladding (Fig. 24.7, bottom). Fibreoptic instruments such as endoscopes use bundles of such flexible fibres to transmit light easily round corners.

A high-intensity light source is used to provide illumination at the end of an endoscope within a patient's body. The light passes from the light source to the endoscope through a fibreoptic light guide which can be coupled to the endoscope. The light source produces heat as well as light and it is possible for a patient to be burnt and surgical drapes to be ignited if the light guide is uncoupled from the endoscope and laid on the patient or the drapes while the light source is still

Figure 24.7 Principle of optical fibres

switched on. The light source should be switched off before the light guide is disconnected from the endoscope, even if the disconnection is for a short time.

Optical fibres may also be used to direct the high-intensity output from lasers to the site where it is needed.

Laser Safety

The effect of lasers on the retina of the eye is used therapeutically as mentioned above. However, the eye is also the organ most at risk when lasers are used, because the beam may be focused by the lens onto the retina and cause irreversible damage in a very short time. Because the carbon dioxide laser beam is absorbed within 200 μm of the tissue surface, this laser is a hazard to the cornea rather than the retina. The laser beam can be accidentally reflected into the eye from a shiny surface such as an operating instrument, so matt surfaces are preferred and well-fitting protective goggles which absorb radiation of the wavelength at which the laser operates should always be worn. Skin protection of personnel is not usually necessary but the patient's tissues adjacent to the lesion to be treated should be protected by water-soaked pads.

A low-power or secondary light beam is used to aim the laser and the operator should only fire the beam of laser radiation when it is correctly aimed. All staff present should be warned when the laser is about to be fired and a special warning sign should be conspicuously displayed outside the door of the operating area (Fig. 24.5B).

The other danger is that a high-power laser beam is capable of igniting flammable materials such as rubber or plastic. Tubes carrying oxygen or anaesthetic gases may be damaged by the laser beam and should be protected by wrapping them with metal tape or damp muslin. Alternatively, special noncombustible laser-resistant tubes have been produced. Local rules for the operation of each laser should be drawn up after discussion with a laser protection adviser.

Magnetic Resonance Imaging

Magnetic resonance imaging (MRI) units produce images of the body in cross section and in three dimensions by detecting the effects of induced changes in the magnetic field of the nuclei of selected elements present in the body.

The nuclei of atoms spin and since nuclei are charged, the spinning charge results, for most nuclei, in a magnetic field, i.e. most nuclei behave like small magnets. In an MRI unit, the magnetic fields of the nuclei within the part of the body to be imaged are aligned by placing this part in a powerful external magnetic field. The nuclei are then turned out of alignment with this magnetic field by applying a short pulse of a magnetic field perpendicular to the main field. The nuclei then precess: i.e. like a gyroscope or a top, they rotate about an axis different from the one about which they are spinning. The precession of the nuclei produces a rotating magnetic field which is measured from the magnitude of the electrical signal induced in a set of coils within the MRI unit. The detected signals are then used to form an image of the body.

After the pulse which induces nuclear precession, the nuclei eventually realign with the main field. The rate at which realignment takes place and the relative importance of the various physical processes which cause the realignment depend on the type of nucleus – i.e. the element and its isotope – and on the molecule of which the element may form a part. This latter dependency occurs because a molecule produces a small magnetic field, which contributes to the total field acting on a particular nucleus, and this varies both with the nature of the molecule concerned and the position of a particular atom within it.

A combination of nonuniform magnetic fields, specific pulse sequences and complex analysis of the resulting nuclear precession allows the determination of the relative abundance of certain elements throughout the body and the display of this information as a cross-sectional image of the body. The principal difficulty is that, for many elements, the signal produced by the nuclear precession is small.

The simplest element to use for imaging purposes is hydrogen, because it is abundant in the body, as one of the constituents of water, and has a strong response to an external magnetic field.

Also of interest is phosphorus, because of its presence in the molecules of ADP and ATP; this allows various metabolic processes to be studied. The nuclear magnetic resonance signal produced by phosphorus in the body is weaker, so a more powerful magnet is needed to produce good-quality images.

Magnetic resonance spectroscopy is a method of determining the relative abundance of a range of substances in in-vitro samples or locally *in vivo*.

Magnet Types

Magnets in use in MRI units have a magnetic flux density generally between 0.2 and 4 tesla.

The very powerful magnetic field present in MRI units may be created either by a permanent magnet or an electromagnet. The disadvantages of permanent magnets compared with electromagnets are, firstly, that the magnetic field cannot be switched off and, secondly, that the magnet is very heavy.

The electromagnets used in MRI units are usually air-cored, i.e. most do not use ferromagnetic cores to increase the magnetic flux density, and the coil current is therefore high. A normal electromagnet can be used up to field strengths of about 0.5 T, but above this value the power dissipated in the windings of the magnet due to the electrical resistance of the conductors produces too much heat. Higher fields must therefore be produced by the use of a superconducting magnet.

Superconductivity

The electrical resistance of certain metals and compounds falls to zero below a transition temperature which is different for individual substances but is typically only a few degrees above 0 K (absolute zero). The coils of MRI units which use superconducting magnets are cooled to below the superconducting transition temperature of the material, such as niobium–titanium alloy, used for the windings. This is achieved by immersion in liquid helium, which boils at 4.2 K at atmospheric pressure. Liquid helium is expensive, so the rate at which it boils off may be further reduced by the use of liquid nitrogen to provide a cooler environment for the liquid helium system.

Safety

The powerful magnetic fields associated with MRI units are able to exert large forces on anything made of ferromagnetic material; furthermore, the AC electromagnetic fields present may induce currents in metallic objects and conductors of all kinds, heating them and producing a rise in temperature locally or throughout the body.

The presence of metallic objects near MRI units, especially ferromagnetic items, is therefore a particular hazard.

Ferromagnetic material may be present inside the body as arterial or aneurysm clips, prostheses, shrapnel, swarf or implanted devices such as pacemakers, all of which could be forced by the magnetic field to move within the body. Such movement and the heating of conducting materials in general could cause tissue damage, perhaps severe enough to cause the death of the patient. Other ferromagnetic material can be accelerated into the field very rapidly, causing injury to anyone in the path of the object or damage to the equipment itself.

Certain body functions can be affected by the strong magnetic field. The body is generally conductive and the movement of blood around the body constitutes a moving conductor. Bodily functions such as this and movements of the body itself can result in the generation of electric potentials and associated currents, as occurs on a smaller scale in, and is the working principle of, the electromagnetic blood flowmeter.

Conversely, naturally occurring potentials and currents such as those produced by the ECG, may be altered as a result of the field. In general, there is the possibility that electric fields generated by the MRI unit can interfere with monitoring equipment and, conversely, electric fields arising in monitoring equipment can degrade the quality of images produced by the MRI unit.

These effects place an upper limit on the field which it is advisable to use and currently this is generally considered to be 2.5–4 T for the whole body.

All these hazards mean that control must be exercised over the personnel having access to the equipment and its immediate vicinity and over the magnetic and electromagnetic field exposure to which individuals are subjected. Safety can be maintained by restricting access to a controlled area or areas inside which the magnetic field is greater than a predefined value. Before entering these controlled areas, everyone must remove from their person all ferromagnetic, metallic and conducting materials and magnetically recorded items such as credit cards. Ferromagnetic objects such as tools, gas cylinders, trolleys, life-support systems, etc., must not be allowed into controlled areas.

Patients with pacemakers must not be examined with MRI equipment and should be kept outside the controlled area.

If anaesthesia is required for a patient who is undergoing MRI, special precautions are necessary to avoid the introduction of metal into the magnetic field of the equipment. Either equipment must be kept out of the controlled area or the equipment must contain no ferromagnetic materials and must be designed for use in the vicinity of MRI units. Thus, anaesthetic equipment constructed entirely of nonferrous materials and using aluminium cylinders is available.

Presentation and Handling of Data and Basic Measurement Concepts

Linear and Nonlinear Scales

The scales on many instrument dials are linear (Fig. 25.1A), but sometimes the scales are nonlinear, being expanded at lower readings to give greater sensitivity. An example is the scale on the oxygen flowmeter of many anaesthetic machines (Fig. 25.1B) in which the conical bore of the interior of the flowmeter is moulded so that low flows of $100-500$ ml min^{-1} register on an expanded scale. This makes adjustment easy both for the low flows used in a closed circuit and for the higher flows used in the Magill system.

A special form of nonlinear scale is the logarithmic type (Fig. 25.1C and D) in which each linear increment on the scale corresponds to a proportionate increase in the amount measured. This scale also has the advantage of allowing greater accuracy when measuring small quantities, while preserving the ability to cover a large range.

Logarithmic Scales

In addition to their use on analogue displays, logarithmic scales are used in digital format to achieve the same advantages of a convenient method of covering a wide range of a quantity. A digital logarithmic scale with 10 as the base can be identified by the exponent or power of 10 as follows:

10^{-3}	10^{-2}	10^{-1}	10^0	10^1	10^2	10^3
0.001	0.01	0.1	1	10	100	1000

One example of the use of a logarithmic scale to the base 10 is pH (Chapter 19), and the use of exponents is considered in Chapter 5. The use of an exponent to the base 10 allows large and small quantities to be presented more compactly and more conveniently than using a large number of digits. Thus, a quantity of 0.00000000251 can be written as 2.51×10^{-9}, and 5,730,000,000 can be expressed as 5.73×10^9.

Many calculators switch automatically into a display indicating the exponent to the base 10 in place of the decimal point when the quantity is too large or too small for the display.

In the SI system, it is recommended that the units are expressed in terms of multiples or submultiples of a thousand (10^3), e.g. kilo (k) for a thousand times and milli (m) for a thousandth. The names and symbols of most of the common multiples in use are given in the Appendix. The multiple is usually chosen so that the numerical value lies within the range 0.1 to 1000; for example:

137,000,000 Pa = 137 MPa
0.002 g = 2 mg

Figure 25.1 Different types of scale

Logarithmic scales are also used in graphs and an example of the use of a semi-logarithmic plot, in which one axis is logarithmic and the other linear, is considered in Chapter 5. A general property of all logarithmic scales is that they do not extend to zero.

Graphical Displays of Data

In circumstances such as the inflation of the lungs by a ventilator, there are several quantities or variables that change in value as inflation proceeds. A list of these variables might include gas flow, airway pressure, alveolar pressure, lung volume and time. Often a change in one variable will affect the value of one or more of the other variables: i.e. the variables are not independent, but the value of one variable is related to or is a function of the value of the others.

A graph is a convenient way of showing how one variable depends on another. It has two axes, each of which is assigned to a variable, and on each axis a scale is marked showing the values taken by that variable. The horizontal axis is called the abscissa or the x-axis and the vertical axis is called the ordinate or the y-axis. Conventionally, the variable that is set, i.e. the independent variable, is assigned to the x-axis and the variable that depends on the value that is set, i.e. the dependent variable, is assigned to the y-axis.

Figure 25.2A illustrates a graph of the way in which inspired volume changes with airway pressure during slow inflation of the lungs in an anaesthetized relaxed patient on a ventilator. In this example, it is assumed that the rate of inflation is so slow that the pressure difference due to the airway resistance can be ignored. Electrical signals of the two variables, volume and pressure, could be obtained by integrating the signal from a pneumotachograph and by a pressure transducer, and the graph could be drawn automatically by an x-y recorder. This type of recorder accepts two electrical inputs for the two variables and plots them simultaneously on a graph. In this example, the volume increases linearly with increasing pressure and the formula which describes the relationship of volume to pressure is:

$$V_I = k_1 P$$

where k_1 is a constant equal to the slope of the graph which, in this case, is V_I/P, the compliance of lungs and chest wall.

If the total volume of air in the lungs is plotted, the graph is modified as shown in Fig. 25.2B and a volume k_2 equal to the functional residual capacity of the lung is added to the inspired volume at each point on the graph as shown.

The formula for the graph then becomes:

$$V_T = k_1 P + k_2$$

Figure 25.2 Linear graphs

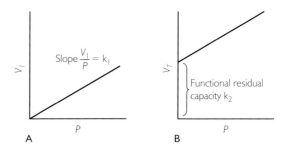

A straight line graph can always be described by an equation of this type. V_T and P are the measured variables in this case, V_T being a function of P; k_1 is the slope or gradient of the graph (in this case the compliance) and k_2 is the intercept on the ordinate or y-axis (in this case the functional residual capacity).

Although k_1 and k_2 are constants, they have different values in different circumstances and in different patients. Such constants are known as parameters. The term parameter is sometimes misused to refer to the variables being measured, but this is best avoided.

Nonlinear Graphs

For practical purposes in turbulent flow (Chapter 2) the following formula describes the relationship between pressure (P) and flow ($\dot{V}$, rate of volume change):

$$P = k\dot{V}^2$$

Figure 25.3A is a graph of this equation and is known as a parabola. A parabola often traces a U shape, as shown in Fig. 25.3B, and may be described in terms of parameters in a similar way to the straight line graph. The general formula for a parabola is

$$y = a + bx + cx^2$$

where y and x are the variables and a, b and c are the parameters.

Other examples of nonlinear graphs are the rectangular hyperbola where $y = k/x$, as exemplified by Boyle's law (Chapter 4), natural exponential functions, e.g. $y = e^{-kx}$ (Chapter 5) and sine waves where $y = k \sin x$ (Chapter 13).

Slope of a Nonlinear Graph

Figure 25.4 shows a graph of the volume expired against time for a rapid expiration. Such a tracing could be obtained with a spirometer (Chapter 3). The slope of

Figure 25.3 Parabolic curves

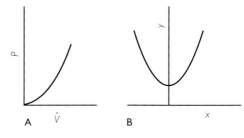

Figure 25.4 Slope of nonlinear graph

the graph at any point represents the expiratory flow at that point and the steepest slope, as shown, is the peak expiratory flow. The slope is obtained by drawing a tangent to the curve.

The slope of any graph of volume against time equals the flow, but it is time-consuming and relatively inaccurate to draw tangents to deduce slope and thus flow. Provided that the equation of the graph is known, a mathematical technique called differentiation may be used to derive the gradient or slope of the graph at any point. Monitors sometimes include electronic processing so that variables can be differentiated if required, e.g. to produce flow from volume change.

Area beneath a Graph

Consider the plot of flow, $\dot{V}$, as a function of time illustrated in Fig. 25.5. This could be produced during an expiration, with a pneumotachograph being used to measure the flow. The area under such a graph equals the product of average flow and time, and so is the volume expired. The shaded area on the graph may be measured by counting squares or by using an instrument known as a planimeter, but the area can also often be deduced mathematically provided the formula for the graph is known. The mathematical process used is known as integration.

Integration may also be used in calculating the area beneath a dye dilution curve in measurements of cardiac output (Chapter 5), and in measurements of the area of a volume–pressure tracing when calculating the work of breathing (Chapter 8). As in the case of differentiation, facilities to integrate variables electronically may be incorporated in monitoring apparatus.

Figure 25.5 Area beneath a graph of flow $\dot{V}$ against time represents volume

Figure 25.6 Pie diagram illustrating distribution of blood flow in the body

Pie Diagram

Graphs are not the only way in which data can be presented diagrammatically, and a pie diagram is a useful technique to illustrate how a certain quantity is divided up. Figure 25.6 illustrates the distribution of the blood flow in the body and gives an immediate impression of the relative importance of the individual organs. The same data could be provided as a table of percentages of blood flow to each organ. However, a pie diagram gives a clearer visual impression of blood flow distribution.

Histogram

In a histogram, the height (or area) of bands or columns is used to illustrate the relative sizes of quantities. In Fig. 25.7, the bands are used to illustrate the relative mean haemoglobin concentrations of adult men and women and could, for example, represent the mean results for several hundred estimations in a laboratory. The histogram gives good visual impact and is particularly useful for illustrations used in teaching. However, in the unmodified form shown, the histogram gives no indication of the range of results, and without additional data, does not prove that the mean haemoglobin of the men is significantly greater than that of the women.

An alternative form of histogram (Fig. 25.8) can be used to illustrate the frequency at which different values of a variable occur. Suppose, for example, that instead of plotting the haemoglobin value as the height of the histogram, the number of men with a given haemoglobin concentration in each 5 g litre^{-1} range is plotted as the height of each band of the histogram. For a survey of 100 fit adult men, the histogram could show a spread of results and, as shown in Fig. 25.8, the histogram traces a bell shape.

Normal Distribution Curve

If haemoglobin values were taken from an even larger population of several thousand and plotted at small increments, then an even smoother bell shape would

Figure 25.7 Histogram illustrating the haemoglobin concentrations of men and women

Figure 25.8 Histogram illustrating the frequency distribution of haemoglobin concentration of a large population of men

result, as shown in Fig. 25.9. In the case of many physiological measurements, the shape of this distribution approaches that of a mathematical curve known as the normal distribution (or Gaussian curve). Such a curve can be described in terms of its mean value, which is also its most frequent result, and by its breadth.

The mean of any set of results is formed by taking the sum of all the individual values and dividing by the number of values, and is often expressed as

$$\text{Mean, } \bar{x} = \frac{\Sigma x_i}{n}$$

where Σ means sum of, x_i is an individual result and n is the number of results.

The breadth of the curve is a measure of the variability of the quantity concerned and a statistical term, standard deviation, often given the symbol σ (sigma), is used as a measure of it.

The standard deviation of any set of results can be found from the formula:

$$\text{Standard deviation, } \sigma = \sqrt{\frac{\Sigma (x_i - \bar{x})^2}{n - 1}}$$

but most modern calculators can produce σ automatically from a set of results.

Suppose this distribution of the haemoglobin concentrations of a large number of men was plotted and was found to be a normal distribution with a mean of 160 g litre^{-1} and a standard deviation of 10 g litre^{-1}. It follows from the shape of the normal distribution that 68% of the men have a haemoglobin between 150 g litre^{-1} and 170 g litre^{-1}, that is, within one standard deviation from the

Figure 25.9 Distribution curve for haemoglobin concentration in men

mean, whereas 95.44% of the men have a haemoglobin between 140 g litre^{-1} and 180 g litre^{-1}. A more commonly used range is 1.96 standard deviations on each side of the mean which includes 95% of the results. This range is known as the 95% confidence range, the limits being known as the 95% confidence limits.

If a result occurs which has a value outside the 95% confidence limits, it belongs to a 5% minority in that population. Put another way, the probability of finding a haemoglobin outside the 95% confidence limits is 5%, which is written $P < 0.05$. The result can then be said to be significant at the 5% level. If $P < 0.01$ the result is significant at the 1% level.

The same concepts and calculation of standard deviation may be applied to other measurements such as temperature, blood pressure, electrolytes and carbon dioxide tension.

Sources of Variability

The variability in a set of results arises from several sources:

- the individuals from whom the measurements are taken
- the sampling or recording techniques used
- the measuring apparatus.

A distribution curve could be drawn for each of these sources to indicate the variability of each (Fig. 25.10), but it is found that the relationship between the total variability in the measured values and that of the component sources depends on the square of the standard deviation, which is known as the variance (σ^2):

$$\sigma_F^2 = \sigma_T^2 + \sigma_S^2 + \sigma_I^2$$

where σ_F^2 is the variance of the final measurement, σ_T^2 is the variance of the total population under study, σ_S^2 is the variance of the measuring or sampling technique and σ_I^2 is the variance of the measuring instrument.

The analysis of the component parts of variability in this way is known as an 'analysis of variance' and, in practice, the sources of variation may be more than the three given in this simple example.

The Normal Range

Many laboratories provide normal ranges of values for various tests. Usually this consists of 95% of the most typical results of a survey of 'normal' individuals and

Figure 25.10 Analysis of variance

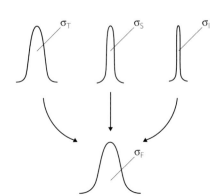

may be expressed as a mean ± 1.96 standard deviations when the distribution approximates to that of a normal distribution. Such a range is known as the 95% confidence interval for the method.

The range includes variability arising from the patients and that from the sampling technique, the time of day at which the sample is drawn and, on some occasions, variation from monthly and annual cycles. The normal range should also include variability from the laboratory's instrument and its use, although this is usually a minor component of total variability for the most common tests.

Instrument Reliability and Quality Control

Although instrument manufacturers provide accuracy ranges for their instruments, larger laboratories include quality control measures to ensure that the precision and accuracy of measurement is maintained in practice. Replicate quality control samples are incorporated into the routine work load and the results compared with those expected, taking into account the precision of the method as assessed from an extensive series of measurements on such samples.

A distinction is made between the terms 'precision' and 'accuracy' when assessing laboratory analysis. Precision is used when referring to the reproducibility of replicate results on a sample within a laboratory. Accuracy is a measure of the difference between the mean of such results and the true value of this material as obtained by the standard method of analysis.

In addition to the inherent variability in the processes of sampling and measuring a variable, it should not be forgotten that occasional gross blunders can occur: examples are incorrect labelling of specimens, a misplaced decimal point or the misuse of reagents or apparatus. A good quality control scheme will check all facets of performance, from patient to report, and not simply the analytical processes.

Variation of the Mean of a Set of Results

If several different sets of results are obtained from a group of patients, the means of each of these sets can be expected to show less variation about the true mean than the individual results themselves. The mean of these means can be calculated and a statistic known as the standard error of the mean is used to indicate the standard deviation of the means in contrast to the standard deviation of the individual results. The standard error of the mean is calculated as follows:

$$\text{Standard error of the mean, SE} = \frac{\sigma}{\sqrt{n}}$$

The standard error of the mean can be used to assess whether a particular set of results has a mean that is significantly different from another set, since confidence limits can be obtained for the mean. The distribution of the means of individual sets of results is generally not a normal distribution: its form depends on the number of results in the set. It is known as the *t*-distribution.

Comparison of Two Sets of Data

Figure 25.11 illustrates the use of confidence limits derived from the standard error of the mean.

On the left of the figure, the mean and 95% confidence limits of the mean for the haemoglobin of a group of 20 men are shown. In the centre of the figure, the

Figure 25.11 Use of the standard error of the mean

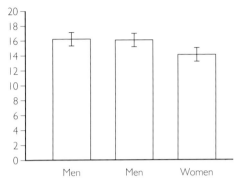

mean and 95% confidence limits for the mean of a different group of 20 men are shown. Since the mean of the first group lies within the confidence limits for the second group, it is unlikely that the means are actually different.

On the right of the figure, the mean and 95% confidence limits for the mean of a group of 20 women are shown. Since the mean of the first group does not lie within the confidence limits for this group, it is likely that the means are actually different.

The Student's t-test may be used to compare two sets of normally distributed samples when the standard errors and means of the two sets are known. The test can be used in either of two forms, depending on whether two separate series of results are being compared (unpaired t-test) or whether results are in the same group of patients (paired t-test). An example of the latter could be a comparison of results before and after treatment.

Modern calculators allow direct calculation of t for unpaired or paired t-tests. The probability that the result is due to chance depends on both the value of t and the number of results and, consequently, tables must be consulted after the value of t is known.

The t-test is commonly used in clinical trials when the measurements have a normal, or near normal, distribution.

Skewed Distribution

Not all measurements show a normal distribution. Figure 25.12A shows a lop-sided or skewed curve. Figure 25.12B illustrates haemoglobin results in a series of women patients in whom anaemia is relatively more frequent than high haemo-globin. It can be seen in each diagram that the most frequently occurring meas-urement, known as the mode, is not the same as the mean. Distribution A has positive skew because the mean occurs at a higher value of the quantity being measured than the mode; distribution B has negative skew.

A distribution may be any shape at all, differing from the normal distribution to a greater extent even than the skewed curves illustrated. It may, for example, have more than one mode. In these circumstances, although a mean and standard deviation can be calculated, the shape of the distribution may be described better by using percentiles. A percentile is the value of the variable being measured which splits the distribution into two parts, with a particular percentage in each. For example, the 17th percentile is the value below which are 17% of the results and above which are 83% of the results. The quartiles divide the results into four equal

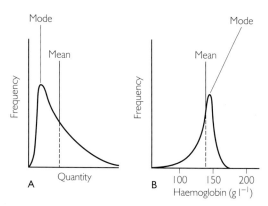

Figure 25.12 Skewed distribution

parts and are therefore the 25th, 50th and 75th percentiles. The 50th percentile or second quartile is known as the median and divides a set of results into two equal parts. The median may therefore be used as an alternative to the mean to indicate the result about which the other results are distributed. The difference between the first and third quartiles is known as the interquartile range and, like the standard deviation, is a measure of the spread of the distribution. An alternative, the semi-interquartile range, is half the interquartile range. The range of a set of results is the difference between the greatest and the least result.

If statistics or tests which are applicable to the normal distribution only are used for non-normal distributions, they may give erroneous results. For example, the 95% confidence limits may not be at 1.96 standard deviations from the mean. Comparison of two sets of results by means of a Student's t-test will also be inappropriate if the distributions deviate greatly from the form of the normal distribution.

There are other statistical techniques which can be used for results that are not distributed normally. These alternative techniques are called nonparametric because they do not assume anything about the parameters of the distributions being compared.

Nonparametric Tests

An example of a nonparametric test is the Wilcoxon rank sum test. It is used to assess whether there is any significant difference between two sets of measurements. Consider the example in Table 25.1, which gives the sleeping time in minutes of 20 patients randomly given different drugs, so that 10 are given drug A and 10 drug B.

The two sets of measurements are ranked: the highest from either set being given the value 1, the next 2, and so on. If two values are identical, the rank figure is averaged as shown. The sum of the ranks for the two sets of measurements can then be calculated. Consultation of tables then shows that the ranking figures 86.5 and 123.5 do not reach significance at the 5% level for the 10 patients concerned in each group.

This example included data from measurements in two different groups of patients. In some experimental trials, two sets of data may be obtained from the same patient. These are known as paired values. The statistical significance of the difference between paired values may be assessed using similar ranking techniques and examples include the Wilcoxon paired test and Spearman's rank test, but full details of these are beyond the scope of this book.

Table 25.1 The Wilcoxon rank sum text			
Sleeping time (min) Drug A	Rank	Sleeping time (min) Drug B	Rank
100	5.5	92	9.5
83	13	78	16
126	1	63	19
65	18	59	20
92	9.5	89	11
81	14	101	4
111	2	76	17
100	5.5	95	7
79	15	94	8
103	3	87	12
940	86.5	834	123.5
mean $\bar{x}_1$, = 94.0		mean $\bar{x}_2$, = 83.4	

Another test is the chi-squared (χ^2) test, in which the frequency of observed results is compared with the expected frequency. This test may be used when assessing the effectiveness of drugs in producing a particular result. If the expected result is regarded as no change, the probability of the obtained result being significant can be assessed. This is often called the null hypothesis.

Scatter Diagrams

When individual results are plotted as points on a graph, they are usually scattered, although an underlying trend may be apparent. A scatter diagram (Fig. 25.13) thus gives an impression of how the results are distributed. The example shows results taken before and after treatment and it is helpful to include a line on the scattergram to indicate the line of identical performance, where $x = y$, as shown. In the example in Fig. 25.13A, all the results are below the line of identical performance and so it is obvious that, despite the variability of the results, the post-treatment measurements were always lower than the pre-treatment values. In Fig. 25.13B, all the results are closely distributed around the line of identical performance and it is apparent that the treatment had no effect.

Regression and Correlation

The line providing the best fit to the points in a scatter diagram is known as a regression line; a measure of how well the points fit the line is the correlation

Figure 25.13 Scatter diagrams illustrating the use of the line of identical performance

A

B

coefficient. The correlation coefficient lies between 0 and 1: a value of 1 indicates perfect agreement between the points and the regression line and a value of 0 indicates no agreement between the points and the line.

A regression line may be linear or curved and it is misleading to fit a linear regression line to a set of points if it is obvious that the points indicate a possible nonlinear relationship or if the scatter is so great that it precludes a decision on whether the relationship is linear or not.

Performance of Predictive Tests

Many tests which are performed in medicine have the object of predicting whether a patient has a certain condition or not. The correctness with which such tests predict the condition can frequently be checked in some other way which it is less convenient or desirable to use regularly, because it is more invasive, for example. Few, if any, of such predictive tests are completely accurate, so in a comparative trial of such a test, a table of the numbers of patients whose conditions were assessed correctly and those whose were not can be drawn up, as shown in Table 25.2.

There are several indicators which show how good the test is and they are defined as follows:

$$\text{Sensitivity} = \frac{\text{True positives}}{\text{True positives} + \text{False negatives}}$$

$$\text{Specificity} = \frac{\text{True negative}}{\text{True negatives} + \text{False positives}}$$

$$\text{Predictive value positive} = \frac{\text{True positives}}{\text{True positives} + \text{False positives}}$$

$$\text{Predictive value negative} = \frac{\text{True negative}}{\text{True negatives} + \text{False negatives}}$$

$$\text{Accuracy} = \frac{\text{True positives} + \text{True negatives}}{\text{Total}}$$

Use of Statistics

Any statistical test is useful only in the appropriate circumstances in a correctly designed experimental trial, and statistical advice should be obtained before the trial begins. The effectiveness of a clinical trial depends on the selection of patients in a truly random but not unethical way, and the exclusion of factors which may obscure the result. It is too late once the trial has been completed to rectify the inadequacy of the design by the use of statistics.

In some cases where one treatment is being compared with another, it is important that the trial is terminated as soon as one treatment is shown to be sig-

Table 25.2 Performance of predictive tests		
	Test does not indicate condition	Test does indicate condition
Condition not present	True negatives	False positives
Condition present	False negatives	True positives

nificantly better than another so that patients do not continue to receive an inferior treatment. Sequential clinical trials are designed so that the trial can be terminated as soon as a significant result is obtained.

Basic Measurement Concepts

The function of a measurement system is to convert the value of some physical quantity to a form which can be observed and recorded. The measurement system has several characteristics that describe how nearly the value that the system displays matches the true value of the quantity being measured.

Linearity

Linearity is a measure of the degree to which the displayed value is proportional to the true value. Figure 25.14 is a graph of the behaviour of a blood pressure transducer: the x-axis is the true blood pressure actually present in the patient's artery and the y-axis is the pressure displayed on the screen of a patient monitor. The solid line shows the ideal behaviour. For the ideal line, at every value of true blood pressure, the displayed value is equal to this true value. The displayed value is proportional to the true value – the proportionality constant in this case being 1.

The dotted line shows the actual behaviour of the transducer. It can be seen that the displayed value is correct when the pressure in the artery is 0 mmHg or 300 mmHg, but at other values the displayed value is different from the true value. The maximum difference, i.e. error, occurs when the true value is 150 mmHg. At this point, the graph shows that the displayed value is 165 mmHg, i.e. 15 mmHg more. So the displayed value is not proportional to the true value. This is also evident from the fact that the dotted line is not straight.

A figure known as the nonlinearity can be used to indicate the degree to which the relationship between a true value and a measured value differs from the ideal. In the example shown in the figure, the nonlinearity is 15 mmHg, but this would more commonly be quoted as ±7.5 mmHg, because adjustment of the transducer response could move the dotted line to the right by 7.5 mmHg. The transducer response would then be 7.5 mmHg too high at the midpoint of the graph and 7.5 mmHg too low at each end of the graph, but less than this at points in between. It is also common practice to express nonlinearity as a percentage of the maximum output. In this case:

$$\text{Nonlinearity} = \frac{\pm 7.5 \text{mmHg}}{300 \text{mmHg}} = \pm 2.5\%$$

The nonlinearity of the graph used for illustration is much greater than would be exhibited by a normal transducer; the effect has been exaggerated for clarity. Real transducers typically have nonlinearities of less than 1%, so the error in the measurement caused by nonlinearity would typically be less than ±1.5 mmHg.

Measurement systems in general are nonlinear, but the nonlinearity is not always apparent when the system is used over a small range. Inspection of Fig. 25.14 shows that the dotted line is more clearly perceived to be curved over the range from 0 to 300 mmHg than over the range 0 to 30 mmHg, for example. Even when nonlinearity is a problem, compensation can often be arranged by electronic means. It is possible to store a table of corrections electronically and to use such a table in monitoring equipment to correct measured values. This technique is used in pulse oximeters, where calibration of the equipment is carried out with

Figure 25.14 Nonlinearity

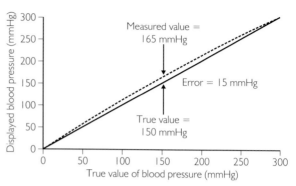

volunteers. The relationship between the measured values derived from the signal received from the pulse oximeter probe and values of haemoglobin saturation is stored in such a table and is then used to select the correct value for display.

Drift

Drift is a measure of the degree to which the displayed value changes over a period of time when the true value is constant. Figure 25.15 illustrates the effect of drift on the performance of a blood pressure measuring system. The solid line represents the ideal response. Suppose the system has this response, but over a period of time the response changes to that represented by the dotted line. At each point over the range of the measuring system, the displayed value is 15 mmHg greater than the true value. The behaviour of the system is still linear, but an offset has been introduced. The system can be restored to a correct response by calibrating the system at one point; all other points will then be correct also.

The dashed line shows drift in which both the offset and the gradient of the line have changed. In this case, calibration at one point will not result in correct performance at all other points. A two-point calibration is required to correct both the offset and the change of gradient.

Drift often occurs as a result of temperature changes as mechanical systems such as the diaphragm of a blood pressure transducer expand and contract. Measuring systems also age; irreversible changes take place in blood gas electrodes, for example. For these reasons, many items of equipment have automatic

Figure 25.15 Drift

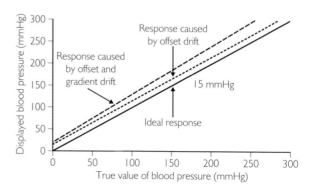

calibration procedures. One-point calibrations may be carried out frequently, perhaps before each measurement, since offset drift develops more quickly, and two or more point calibrations may be carried out at less frequent intervals to correct gradient drift.

Hysteresis

Hysteresis is a measure of the difference in the displayed value for a given true value when the true value is increasing compared to when it is decreasing. Figure 25.16 illustrates hysteresis.

The solid line shows the behaviour of the system while the true value is increasing; the dotted line shows the behaviour while the true value is decreasing. It can be seen that for a given true value, the displayed value depends on whether the true value is increasing or decreasing. In practice, the situation is somewhat more complex than represented by the graph because the pressure does not usually vary between the extremes of the range. A system in which the pressure varies between 120 mmHg and 80 mmHg, for example, will exhibit a smaller version of the curve shown, so that the effect of hysteresis is less. Fortunately, hysteresis is rarely a serious problem in monitoring applications in medicine.

Static and Dynamic Response

The graphs of linearity, drift and hysteresis discussed previously illustrated the behaviour of the measuring system when the measured values were not changing, i.e. when the system was in equilibrium. The response of a measuring system in equilibrium is the static response. The behaviour of a measuring system when the measured value is changing, as it often is in monitoring systems, is known as the dynamic response and can be different from the static response. The dynamic response of many measuring systems used in medicine is one of three types.

Zero-order response

In a measuring system with zero-order response, the displayed value tracks the value that is being measured immediately. An example of a zero-order response is the position control or gain control of a patient monitor. The display responds immediately to adjustment of the control.

Figure 25.16 Hysteresis

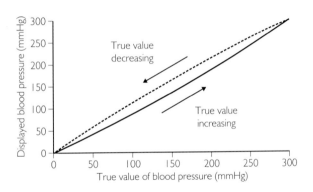

Figure 25.17 First order response

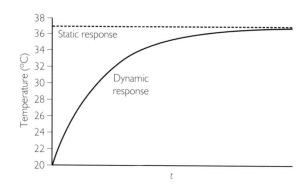

First-order response

In a measuring system with first-order response, the displayed value approaches the value that is being measured in an exponential manner. An example of a first-order system is a temperature probe. Figure 25.17 is a graph of the temperature indicated by a patient monitor connected to a temperature probe which has been attached to a patient. The probe was initially at room temperature (20°C), but its temperature increased when it was attached to the patient, whose temperature was 37°C. The temperature of the probe approached the temperature of the patient asymptotically. In equilibrium (the static response), the probe registered 37°C.

Second-order response

In a measuring system with second-order response, the behaviour is more complex. The response may resemble that of a first-order system or may oscillate about the true value. An example of a second-order system is the measurement of arterial blood pressure with a pressure transducer. The problems of resonance and damping associated with second-order response are discussed briefly in Chapter 17.

Assessment of Awareness during Anaesthesia

Depth of Anaesthesia

The state of anaesthesia has proved to be difficult to define, but certain features would be agreed widely. The major concern of the patient is to remain oblivious of any events during surgery and to recover with minimum discomfort after the procedure. Considerable distress may be caused to patients who are completely aware and who experience pain during surgery. Reports from patients who have suffered this experience provide a dramatic insight into the trauma involved.

Awareness during anaesthesia may not be identifiable from the observation of cardiovascular data but may cause major psychological trauma during surgery and lead to longer-term effects such as mental depression, personality transformation and sleep disturbances including dreams, nightmares and insomnia. In addition, it may not be simple to detect that patients were aware during general anaesthesia from postoperative questioning of the patient.

There is no agreed standard available against which any technique to measure depth of anaesthesia can be judged. However, any measure of anaesthetic depth should be able to provide sufficient information to enable satisfactory general anaesthesia to be produced during surgery. The closest control of anaesthesia is required when the patient is breathing spontaneously during surgery since excessively light anaesthesia leads to the patient moving, whereas excessively deep anaesthesia results in depression of respiration.

Requirements for satisfactory anaesthesia are

- adequate cardiovascular and respiratory stability
- ideally no, or at least only minimal, patient movement
- no awareness or recall of events during the procedure
- similar values for different types of anaesthetic agents at equipotent doses
- values at recovery from anaesthesia similar to those obtained before induction
- appropriate change during surgical stimulation
- unaffected by alterations in the cardiovascular system or by cardioactive drugs
- marked difference in the signal between consciousness and unconsciousness.

These conditions are part of the standard against which any monitor of the depth of anaesthesia can be judged.

Simple Techniques for Assessing Anaesthetic Depth

Clinical Signs

Most anaesthetists control the administration of anaesthetic agents by observing clinical signs, although these do not always provide an accurate assessment. After the start of surgery, the anaesthetist is guided usually by the patient's residual autonomic and somatic responses.

Respiratory and Skeletal Muscle Activity

Frequency and depth of respiration are useful indicators of anaesthetic adequacy during spontaneous respiration and any skeletal muscle response in relation to surgical stimulation indicates insufficient anaesthesia. However, these signs are lost in a paralysed patient and other observations are then required.

Isolated Forearm Technique

A pneumatic cuff is placed on the patient's upper arm and inflated above systolic pressure before administration of the neuromuscular blocking agent. The lower arm is therefore not paralysed and this allows the anaesthetist to assess the patient's depth of anaesthesia by asking direct questions concerning the sensation of awareness or pain. The patient responds by squeezing the anaesthetist's hand. In this way, obeying the command indicates awareness with possible recall. Spontaneous movement of the patient's isolated arm may interfere with this technique and the duration of pneumatic cuff inflation must be limited. This technique has therefore been restricted to research studies.

Stability of the Sympathetic Nervous System

The PRST scoring system was developed to provide an unbiased assessment of the degree of sympathetic stimulation. A score is allocated to each variable and a total PRST score calculated based on four variables:

- systolic arterial Pressure
- pulse Rate
- Sweating
- Tear formation.

Arterial pressure and heart rate are probably the most commonly used signs to indicate the level of general anaesthesia, but there is considerable evidence that these measurements are of limited value in predicting which patients will be aware or not. Sweat production and tear formation may also be considered as indicators of the degree of sympathetic activity during surgery. However, the PRST scoring system has not been shown in controlled trials to provide any real benefit in detecting awareness and there are many reports where simple clinical signs have failed to guarantee lack of awareness.

Value of Clinical Signs

Clinical signs are used by most anaesthetists to control the administration of hypnotic and analgesic drugs. Where muscle relaxants have not been administered, patient movement is probably the most important clinical sign and can be taken to indicate an inadequate level of anaesthesia. It should be remembered that the minimum alveolar concentration (MAC) of a volatile anaesthetic is the concentration at which 50% of patients make a gross, purposeful movement in response to surgical stimulation but there is no report of patient recall of the event. However, when relaxants have been administered, movement is lost as a sign of inadequate anaesthesia and reliance must be placed on indirect signs of the patient's arousal. The frequency of awareness with recall during surgical anaesthesia has been reported to be about 2 per 1000 cases over the past 10 years.

Analysis of the EEG

In the electroencephalogram, the EEG, electrodes are positioned around the patient's head to record the characteristic potentials arising from the activity of the cerebral cortex. The potentials are much smaller than those of the electrocardiogram (ECG), being only about 50 µV. The appearance of the EEG wave pattern is also important. For example, slow, low-frequency waves may indicate cerebral hypoxia. Deepening the level of anaesthesia is usually accompanied by a decrease in the frequency and amplitude of the EEG.

Burst Suppression

Burst suppression of the EEG occurs at a deep level of anaesthesia. A burst of electrical activity is followed by a period during which there is relatively little activity (Fig. 26.1).

However, analysis of the standard EEG is too complex for routine use in anaesthesia, so alternative techniques have been developed.

Figure 26.1 Burst suppression of the EEG

Compressed Spectral Array

The compressed spectral array (CSA), illustrated in Fig. 26.2, represents an attempt to analyse the raw EEG data to produce a simplified analysis of brain activity. Discrete time periods of EEG activity, such as 8 s, are recorded and then subjected to fast Fourier transformation (see Chapter 13), which calculates the total power contained within different frequencies. The power in the different frequencies may be displayed graphically as a series of troughs and peaks and, under anaesthesia, power shifts to the lower frequencies and provides a guide to the extent of cerebral suppression.

More complex EEG processing attempts to extract single numbers from the CSA and some of these numbers have been used in the assessment of anaesthetic depth. Two have been assessed for clinical significance: spectral edge frequency and median frequency.

The spectral edge is the frequency below which is contained 95% of the total power in the CSA and it provides a measure of the upper edge of the power spectrum. A progressive reduction in this value has been demonstrated with increasing concentrations of anaesthetic agents. However, this does not appear to be a satisfactory technique to assess anaesthetic depth since during the transition from deep to light levels of anaesthesia, the relationship between spectral edge and drug concentration is poor.

The median frequency represents the midpoint of the power distribution in the CSA and is the frequency below and above which lies 50% of the total power in the EEG. It has been suggested that the median frequency is a more accurate indicator of depth of anaesthesia than spectral edge in that median frequency appears to have a closer relationship with drug concentrations in both the uptake and elimination phases. However, varying patterns of CSA are obtained when patients are anaesthetized with different types of anaesthetic agents.

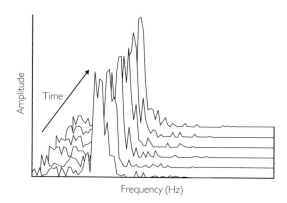

Figure 26.2 Compressed spectral array

Bispectral Analysis

Bispectral analysis is a more recent method of EEG analysis based on the phase and power relationships between the different frequencies present in the EEG. In contrast, when the compressed spectral array is calculated, any information concerning the phase relationship of the different waves is discarded. Bispectral analysis uses a mathematical calculation to quantify the relationship between frequency triplets present in the EEG. The frequency triplets are any two frequencies, f_1 and f_2, and the sum of those frequencies, $f_1 + f_2$. When the analysis has been performed, a bispectrum, which is a function of the two frequencies f_1 and f_2, results. The bispectrum contains the phase and power relationships between any two frequencies in the EEG.

From the bispectrum, a measure of the phase relationship between the frequency triplets, known as the bicoherence, can be calculated. The bicoherence is a value between 0 and 1. If the phase relationships between the frequencies in a triplet tend to be random, the biocoherence approaches 0. Conversely, if the phase differences between the frequencies tend to be fixed, the bicoherence approaches 1.

In the EEG, independent generation of different frequencies tends to produce a low value of bicoherence. The bicoherence tends to increase as depth of anaesthesia increases.

Bispectral Index (BIS) Technique

The BIS is a commercially available system which calculates a weighted average of spectral array, bicoherence and burst suppression parameters that analyse the phase and frequency relationships among the component frequencies in the EEG. The BIS has proved more reliable than other types of analysis such as the compressed spectral array, but may still suffer from some degree of variability when using different types of anaesthetic agents.

Entropy

Entropy quantifies the disorder in a system and characterizes the complexity of a signal. Analysis techniques based on measures of entropy are being assessed for their value in distinguishing between different levels of sedation and hypnosis.

Figure 26.3 Auditory evoked potential: (A) conscious, (B) under anaesthesia

(a)   (b)

Evoked Potentials

A further development of EEG monitoring is the use of the evoked potential (EP), which is also known as the event-related potential (ERP) or evoked response (ER). The evoked potential is produced when a person receives a peripheral stimulus, which may be somatosensory, auditory or visual. Since the evoked potential is only a few microvolts in amplitude, it is masked by the general electrical activity which constitutes the EEG. To obtain the EP, it is necessary to repeat the stimulus many times and average the EEG obtained during a fixed period following each stimulus. The average background EEG amplitude in the resulting waveform is then *decreased* because the EEG is not related to the stimulus. The average EP amplitude is *increased* because its activity is related in time to the stimulus. Examination of evoked potentials may be used to check that neurological pathways are not injured during specialized surgery, but meticulous care is required both in the use of the system and in interpretation of the results.

Auditory Evoked Potentials

As depth of anaesthesia increases, evoked potentials diminish. The auditory evoked potential is one of the last of these potentials to disappear and it is therefore useful as an indication of whether a patient is fully anaesthetized (Fig. 26.3). The auditory evoked potential has been shown to correlate well with depth of anaesthesia produced by either inhalational or intravenous anaesthesia. A patient's auditory system is stimulated by means of clicks applied at a rate of 5–10 per second through headphones to both ears of a patient. The evoked potential is obtained by recording the EEG from electrodes attached to the mastoid and forehead, recording taking place during a period of 80–150 ms after each click. The EEG signal is amplified and the evoked potential extracted by averaging several hundred or thousand individual responses. The averaging process removes the random, background electrical activity and leaves only the evoked potential, which is correlated in time to the stimulating clicks.

The auditory steady-state response is a technique in which the sound stimuli are administered at a frequency of about 40 Hz. The amplitude of the EEG response has been investigated in relationship to the loss of and recovery from consciousness. The results of this technique are not yet conclusive.

Appendix

Units of Measurement

The Système International d'Unités or SI system was introduced in 1960. As this is the system generally used in this book, a resumé is provided.

Base SI Units

There are seven base units in the SI system from which all other units are derived. The base units are as follows with the symbol for the unit given in brackets:

1. *Length*: metre (m)
   The metre is the distance light travels in a specified fraction of a second.
2. *Mass*: kilogram (kg)
   The kilogram is based on the mass of a 1 kilogram prototype held at Sèvres near Paris.
3. *Time*: second (s)
   The second is based on the frequency of radiation emitted from caesium-133.
4. *Current*: ampere (A)
   The ampere is the current which produces a force of 2×10^{-7} newtons per metre between two conductors 1 metre apart in a vacuum.
5. *Temperature*: kelvin (K)
   The kelvin is 1/273.16 of the thermodynamic temperature of the triple point of water. (The triple point is the point at which water vapour, ice and liquid water are in equilibrium.)
6. *Luminous intensity*: candela (cd)
   The candela is based on the luminous intensity of a perfect radiating black body at a specified high temperature.
7. *Amount of substance*: mole (mol)
   The mole is the amount of substance which contains as many elementary particles as there are atoms in 0.012 kg of carbon-12.

Derived Units

From these seven base units, numerous derived units may be obtained. Examples of some of the more important are as follows:

Temperature: degree Celsius (°C)
The size of the degree Celsius is identical to the kelvin and the relationship is:

$$°C = K - 273.15$$

Force: newton (N)

A force of 1 newton will give a mass of 1 kilogram an acceleration of 1 metre per second per second.

$$1 \text{ N} = 1 \text{ kg m s}^{-2}$$

Pressure: pascal (Pa)

A pascal is the pressure of 1 newton per square metre.

$$1 \text{ Pa} = 1 \text{ N m}^{-2}$$

Pressure: bar (bar)

A bar is 100 kilopascals. It is not an SI unit, but has been retained for general use.

Energy: joule (J)

A joule is the energy expended when the point of application of a force of 1 newton moves 1 metre in the direction of the force.

$$1 \text{ J} = 1 \text{ Nm}$$

Energy: electronvolt (eV)

The electronvolt (eV) is used for certain types of electromagnetic radiation. An electron volt is the energy required to move one electron through a potential difference of one volt in a vacuum and is approximately equal to 1.6×10^{-19} J.

Power: watt (W)

Power is the rate of energy expenditure. One watt is 1 joule per second.

$$1 \text{ W} = 1 \text{ J s}^{-1}$$

Frequency: hertz (Hz)

One hertz is a frequency of 1 cycle per second.

Volume: cubic metre (m^3)

Volume: litre (l)

The official SI unit of volume is the cubic metre (m^3), but the litre, one-thousandth of a cubic metre, is a permitted unit for general use.

$$1 \text{ litre} = 10^{-3} \text{ m}^3$$

Electrical Units

The main units used in this book are:

Potential: volt (V)

One volt is the difference of electrical potential between two points of a conductor carrying a constant current of 1 ampere, when the power dissipated between these points is 1 watt.

$$V = W \text{ A}^{-1}$$

Resistance: ohm (Ω)

If a potential of 1 volt is applied across a conductor and produces a current of 1 ampere, the resistance of this conductor is 1 ohm.

$$\Omega = V \text{ A}^{-1}$$

Charge: coulomb (C)

One coulomb is the quantity of electricity transported in 1 second by a current of 1 ampere.

$$C = A \text{ s}$$

Capacitance: farad (F)
A capacitor has one farad of capacitance if a potential difference of 1 volt is present across its plates, when a charge of 1 coulomb is held by them.

$$F = C\, V^{-1}$$

Units not in the SI System

Several unofficial units are still in common use:

Pressure: millimetres of mercury (mmHg)
It should be noted that 1 kilopascal is equivalent to approximately 7.5 mmHg and 1 bar is therefore 750 mmHg.

Pressure: centimetres of water (cmH_2O)
One centimetre of water pressure is approximately 98 Pa. (1 kPa = 10.2 cmH_2O.)

Pressure: standard atmosphere (atm)
A standard or normal atmosphere is the pressure of 101.325 kPa. A bar is therefore about the same as an atmosphere.

Energy: calorie (cal)
A calorie is 4.18 J. Calorie spelt with a capital 'C' may represent 1000 calories when it is used in dietary nutrition.

Force: kilogram weight (kg wt)
The kilogram weight, sometimes called the kilopond, is the force of gravity on a mass of 1 kilogram. Gravity gives an acceleration of 9.81 m s^{-2}: consequently,

$$1 \text{ kilogram weight} = 9.81 \text{ N}$$

Multiples of Units

In the SI system, the preferred multiples of the units are in terms of a thousand and the commoner multiples and their symbols (in brackets) are as follows:

pico 10^{-12} (p)

nano 10^{-9} (n)

micro 10^{-6} (μ)

milli 10^{-3} (m)

kilo 10^{3} (k)

mega 10^{6} (M)

giga 10^{9} (G)

Standard Temperature and Pressure (STP)

When expressed in SI units, STP is 273.15 K (0°C) and 101.325 kPa.

Index

Page numbers followed by f indicate figures.